Intermittent Fasting for Women Over 50:

Discover How to Lose Weight Fast, Increase Your Energy and Age – Well, Thanks to Intermittent Fasting!

NORA DAVIES

TABLE OF CONTENTS

Introduction

Congratulations on purchasing *Intermittent Fasting for Women Over 50: Discover How to Lose Weight Fast, Increase Your Energy and Age – Well, Thanks to Intermittent Fasting!* and thank you for doing so.

The following chapters will discuss every detail about intermittent fasting, and the major focus will be how it affects women over the age of 50. What most people don't understand is the body of a man and woman are not the same and so their nutritional requirements are also not the same as well. So, the effect of intermittent fasting on a man does not necessarily have to be the same in the case of a woman. But in this book, you will see everything from the perspective of women over the age of 50. Now, I reckon that you have been long searching for ways to deal with the problems of old age and also stay fit. Well, intermittent fasting can be the solution to everything if practiced in the right way.

Firstly, I would like to welcome all of you to this exciting journey of intermittent fasting, and I assure you that if you remain consistent, then you are going to reap the benefits. In this book, I will not only educate you on the why's and how's of intermittent fasting but I have also included some actionable tips and common mistakes at the end of this book. I am researched on this subject and I have myself benefitted a lot from intermittent fasting. So, now, I want everyone to benefit from the knowledge that I have gained over the years.

There are plenty of books on this subject on the market, thanks again for choosing this one! Every effort was made to ensure it is full of as much useful information as possible; please enjoy and if you will find it beneficial please leave a review.

Chapter 1: What Is Intermittent Fasting?

There are different types of diets that you will hear about in today's world. But intermittent fasting is not any diet. It is more like an eating pattern where you have a fasting phase and an eating phase. Both these phases alternate with each other after regular intervals. In this chapter, you will learn in-depth about what intermittent fasting is and what benefits it provides. The best thing about intermittent fasting probably is the fact that it does not have any strict restrictions on what you can and cannot eat. The stress is laid more on the time you are eating and fasting. But most books will tell you about intermittent fasting with respect to men. However, for women, the effects of intermittent fasting are not the same, and so in this book, I have explained how intermittent fasting is going to be beneficial for a woman's body especially those who are over the age of 50.

Types of Intermittent Fasting

The approach to intermittent fasting is not singular, and thus, there are different ways in which you can do it. Also, you need to understand that if you decide to perform intermittent fasting, you don't necessarily have to stick to just a single type. What you can do is try them out or study them in detail and then decide which of them will suit you the best and also can be well incorporated in your lifestyle without any hassle. None of these types are less than the other. All of them have been proved to be beneficial and there is evidence worldwide. There are some famous personalities who can vouch for the method they had followed.

What I would advise you is that don't just stick to any single method. You will have to try your hand at different methods. Try as many of them as possible. It is true that when you read about some of the methods they would not seem much attractive or enticing at first, but you might end up liking them once you try them in real life. So, don't leave out any of the options because your experience with any of the methods might not match with someone else's. Everyone does not respond to this eating pattern in the same manner. This is mostly because of the differences in lifestyle choices and also because of different health criteria. People who are physically active might not have the same exact response to any particular form of fasting as that of those people who are not that active.

Now, coming to your eating window, you can eat anything you want, but that does not mean consuming unhealthy and processed foods. You can have anything that is healthy. Intermittent fasting does not really put that much focus on the meals themselves but rather on the timing of your eating and fasting window. Also, I would advise you not to overdo your meals in the eating window. Eat normally. Some people, especially beginners, tend to overdo their meals just because they had been fasting. Eating more food or more calories than you usually do neutralizes the effect of the fast and so you will not be able to enjoy the added benefits.

There is another thing to keep in mind that is intermittent fasting does not mean you cannot have water or coffee during the fast. It is not a dry fast. You can have these liquids. On the contrary, in the case of dry fasts, people are prohibited from drinking any kind of liquids too. And this includes water as well. But in the case of intermittent fasting, there is no such rule. In fact, there are people who even resort to supplements that are low in calories during their fasting window.

If you want to start with intermittent fasting, and if you are really serious with it, then try to stick to a low-carb diet, and it is going to help you a lot. So that when you are in your eating window, you are restricting the consumption of any extra amount of carbs. So, even if you are eating, your body is not actually completely done with ketosis. Now, this brings me to the next point and that is – the keto diet is one of the best diets that you can follow in intermittent fasting because it promotes the process of ketosis. In a keto diet, you will be consuming low-carb foods that are rich in fat (good fat). This also helps to maintain a state of fat-burning phase in your body.

The 16/8 Method

This is one of the most popular methods of intermittent fasting, and it requires you to perform a fast every day. The fasting period is approximately sixteen hours. For beginners, this is considered to be the best method of intermittent fasting and if you are successful in following it, then your eating window in a day will be reduced to eight hours only. Now, within this eight-hour eating window, fitting two to three meals is not that tough. One of the best ways to perform this fast is to skip your breakfast. And for this, you will have to stop yourself from eating anything after you have completed your dinner.

This means that you will have your first meal at noon the next day. For this, your dinner should have been completed by 8 pm. This means you have to take a light supper. On the contrary, if you prefer having your supper at around 6 pm, then you can consider your supper to be the last meal and then the next day, you can start it earlier. Your first meal can then be at 10 am. The times of eating will strictly vary from one person to another depending on individual lifestyles and schedules of work.

But no matter what your eating and fasting window is, in this method, it is best that you fix the fasting window around your sleeping window. When you are asleep, you will not be eating anything, and so the fast becomes easier. In short, your fasting time coincides with your sleeping time and this is helpful on so many levels, especially for beginners who have just started fasting. Also, in case you do not like the idea of skipping breakfast and sleep for eight hours every day, then you should adjust your fasting time accordingly so that you can have your first meal right after you wake up. In short, adjust your fasting window to end right after you wake, whatever may be your sleeping window, so that you do not have to deal with any discomfort related to hunger when you start the day.

Martin Berkhan, who is a fitness expert, is the person who popularized the 16/8 method of fasting. A typical eating plan would look something like this –

- Breakfast at 12 pm
- Second Meal at 4 pm
- Last Meal at 8 pm

If you are someone who performs regular workouts on a professional level with weights or even normal cardio, then you need to adjust your eating window based on your availability. For example, if you plan to go to the gym or work out at around noon, then you can plan your first meal of the day before that. It should be light, and then it can be your pre-workout meal. And suppose you come back from a workout at around 1 pm, then you can have the biggest meal then.

The 5:2 Diet

In this type of intermittent fasting, your normal eating window will continue for five days in a particular week, and then you will have to restrict your calories on the remaining two days. The calorie intake, at an average, for those two days of the week, should be approximately 500. It is advised that women should not consume more than 500 calories but for men, this value is stretched to 600. If you ask me, then I would say that the best way in which you can make this a success is to have only two meals in a day and each one of them should be around 250 calories each.

Recently, the 5:2 diet has gained quite a momentum among women because you get a lot of flexibility with it. Yes, you have to fast, but it will only be for two days a week. So, people who are really busy in their lives find this method way easier than the others because scheduling becomes easier. One of the ways in which you can accomplish this is not going on lunch dates with your friends on the days when you decide to fast. But there is also a rule that you must follow. The days that you are fasting must not be successive or one after the other. There must be at least a one-day gap in between. Keeping all these things in mind, the days on which most people choose to fast are Mondays and Thursdays. But you can also choose Tuesdays and Thursdays if that is something that is suitable for you.

Also, just like the 16/8 method, here too you should keep in mind that you cannot consume highly calorific foods or go out of your way to consume more food than what you usually do. It is good that you are fasting, but you don't have to overcompensate for it. Unhealthy and carb-heavy meals are a big no at all times.

A 24-Hour Fast

This method is also popularly known as the Eat-Stop-Eat method, where you have to perform a fast for a whole day. It can be tough for beginners but it is not impossible. It is somewhat close to the concept of the 5:2 diet but the only difference is that you are not consuming food at all when you are performing a 24-hour fast. Brad Pilon, who is a fitness expert, is the person responsible for introducing this method of intermittent fasting among the masses.

Let me give you an example of this fast. For example, you have your dinner at 7 pm today, and that is when your fast begins. You are not going to have anything after that and break your fast at dinner again the next day at 7 pm. This is how a 24-hour fast looks like. Just like the other fasts, you are allowed to drink coffee and water but not anything else. The timings can be adjusted to whatever is suitable for you. You can do it from lunch to lunch or even from breakfast to breakfast. But mind it, you can get bad cravings if you are new to this and don't let them trick you into having large meals in your eating window.

Alternate Day Fasting

In this method of intermittent fasting, you will be fasting every alternate day. One day you will be eating the way you do, and then the next day you will be fasting. The day after that will be your eating day and the cycle continues like this. This method of intermittent fasting is considered to be one of the better and more advanced methods to do this process. And experts do not advise this particular method for beginners at all. Before you move on to an advanced method like this one, it is advisable that you start off with smaller fasting windows.

In this type of fast, when you are in your fasting window, you will have to perform a complete twenty-four hours fast. The rules are the same for this one as well. You can drink coffee and water, but no food item is allowed. The difference with the Eat-Stop-Eat method is that in the case of alternate-day fasting, you will be performing two to three of full fasting whereas, in the former method, it is only one day a week. But again, never overcompensate with food; otherwise, all this fasting will be of no use to your health.

The Warrior Diet

In this type of intermittent fasting, you will be fasting every day, but the only difference is that you will take one meal at the end of the day that is large. But throughout the day, you will not have any food except for coffee or water. On the other hand, the Warrior Diet has several other variations where the intake of certain fruits and raw veggies is allowed during the fasting window. Also, if you are not aware of this, then the Warrior Diet was actually one of the very first methods of intermittent fasting that became popular. The type of dishes that you can have in this type of diet coincides with that of the Paleo Diet.

Spontaneous Meal Skipping

If you don't like the idea of following a schedule and planning so much for starting intermittent fasting, then you can try out the spontaneous meal skipping method. This method aims at helping people realize the benefits of intermittent fasting by skipping meals whenever they feel like doing so. For example, if you are not a breakfast kind of person, then you can skip it and then have your next meal at lunch. But no matter which meal you skip, don't forget that you cannot overdo the next meal you have.

Benefits of Intermittent Fasting

Now that more and more people are trying out the concept of intermittent fasting, they have come to realize the several benefits that this particular eating pattern has. There are, of course, some general benefits like restrictions in calories which lead to weight loss. Also, since you do not have to make certain meals in a day, it will save your time and also reduce effort on an everyday basis. Also, if you follow intermittent fasting by skipping breakfast every day, then you are actually saving up on the expenses that are required to make breakfast. There is another advantage to it, and that is – you do not have to wake up early in the morning to make your breakfast and you can either sleep a bit more or utilize the time for other activities. But apart from what I have already mentioned here, there are several other benefits associated with intermittent fasting and they are as follows.

Weight Loss

The major reason why people start intermittent fasting is that they want to shed some weight, and with intermittent fasting, it is definitely possible. So, if you are able to execute it properly, then the number of meals you consume in a day will become lower. Thus, the overall intake of calories in a day automatically falls below the usual number. But there is another way in which intermittent fasting helps in weight loss and that is by regulating hormone function. Now, you must be wondering what exactly happens.

Well, for starters, intermittent fasting promotes the levels of growth hormones and also helps in reducing the levels of insulin. Along with this, the levels of norepinephrine also rise. The process of breakdown of fat in your body is assisted by the cumulative effect of all these hormonal changes.

That is why it has been noticed that if a person goes for short-term fasting, then his/her metabolic rate increases by as much as fourteen percent. In simpler terms, it means that on a regular basis, burning calories will become easier and greater in number than before. So, if you prefer keeping a count of the calories consumed in a day, then too intermittent fasting is the perfect fit for you. When you are doing it, you are literally forced to consume lesser food and thus, there is an intake of fewer calories which, in turn, boosts your metabolic rate. This again leads to faster burning of calories. So, this is how intermittent fasting is so effective for losing weight.

Lowers Inflammation

There are so many chronic diseases that occur as a result of inflammation, and these are Alzheimer's disease, dementia, and so on. There is one type of inflammation that is necessary. This is when white blood cells shield you against diseases by keeping away viruses and bacteria. But in some cases, like arthritis, the inflammatory response in your body is triggered but in reality, there is no such severe threat at that time. What happens is that the tissues in your body suffer damage due to the autoimmune diseases which create a situation where the body thinks that it is protecting itself from a virus when there is no virus at all.

But, when you are performing intermittent fasting, a certain state is induced in your body known as autophagy. This is the body's process of eliminating damaged and old cells by killing them. Yes, it might sound macabre to you, but it is a very essential process. Think of it like this – your body tries to remove all the old and unwanted particles from your body through this process. The process is very simple and it falls under the body's process of repairing itself. Inflammation is triggered in your body due to these old cells but when autophagy starts, inflammation is reduced.

Ensures Overall Fitness

There is a myth about intermittent fasting that it somehow interferes with the fitness levels of those who perform physical workouts. Some people think that it might lead to a deterioration of their fitness levels. But this is not true, and it has been proven by several studies like the one published in the Journal of Sports Sciences that intermittent fasting does not impact in any negative manner even if you are into regular physical workouts. But what you have to do is you need to reduce your consumption of carbs and also take enough sleep. In fact, your body will show a far better metabolic adaptation if you are into physical training and performing intermittent fasting at the same time.

So, if you think about the long run, then having a better metabolic adaption means that you will reap better benefits and enhance your overall performance. Moreover, when you have a meal after your workout and if you were fasting prior to that then your body's response to that meal would be even better. Your body will show faster and better absorption of nutrients from the post-workout meals. Moreover, you will get better muscle gains if you schedule your fasts properly and maintain a proper diet along with a regular dose of exercise.

Helps in Burning Fat

According to the studies, it is believed that carbs are not a very good source of energy as compared to fats. When you consider the per gram calculation, fats will give you far more energy than carbs. This is also one of the reasons how your hunger can be controlled even when you are performing a low-carb diet. Moreover, during the energy-burning reactions, there are lesser chances of the formation of free radicals if the energy is derived from fats. If you do not know then here is a fact – one of the causes of inflammation is the formation of free radicals in your body. These free radicals lead to the formation of oxidative stress, which is not at all good for your body. Several neurodegenerative diseases happen because of the presence of these free radicals.

When you are into intermittent fasting, there is a product derived from fats known as ketones, and your brain will be prompted to use ketones as a source of energy. This is a better alternative than sugar because ketones are not only efficient but also a much cleaner form of fuel, especially when it comes to your brain.

Increase in the Levels of Energy

Mitochondrial biogenesis and neurogenesis are both promoted when you perform intermittent fasting. The formation of new nerve tissues and brain cells is a process that happens during neurogenesis. Similarly, the formation of new mitochondria happens during mitochondrial biogenesis. When there are more mitochondria in your brain, you will have more power in your brain, and so in the long run, you will not feel lethargic. Instead, you will be more focused on your work and feel full of energy.

Reduces the Risk of Type 2 Diabetes

If you have a family history of type 2 diabetes, then you are obviously at risk of developing it too, but if you perform intermittent fasting, then you can reduce this risk. Moreover, over the past years, one of the major problems that trouble mankind is type 2 diabetes. People develop insulin resistance and that, in turn, leads to higher levels of sugar in the blood. In order to reduce this level, you have to improve your condition of insulin resistance.

It has been noticed that if a person performs intermittent fasting, then they can effectively reduce their levels of fasting blood sugar by four to six percent and the levels of insulin in the fasting stage by 21-30%. Moreover, the major complication that every patient of type 2 diabetes faces is the damage to kidneys, and with intermittent fasting, you can prevent that too. So, not only are you protected from being at a greater risk of developing type 2 diabetes but you are also protected from the risks that come with it.

Enhances Heart Health

Yes, you have heard me right. Intermittent Fasting does help in improving heart conditions. Heart diseases are currently very much prevalent and are the reason for the deaths of so many people on a daily basis. But with intermittent fasting, you will see a positive development in the levels of LDL cholesterol, blood triglycerides, inflammatory markers, blood pressure, and also blood sugar, all of which contribute to the development of heart problems and lowering these means that you are keeping heart problems at bay.

Lesser Cravings

Cravings can be very hard to deal with and are one of the major reasons why people give up on their weight loss regime. The reason behind having such cravings is your disrupted levels of insulin. But when you are performing intermittent fasting, you can effectively keep your insulin levels in check and also work on improving your body's insulin resistance. When your body has gradually adjusted to the situation, there will be lesser production of insulin, and all those sugar cravings will not happen like before.

13

Chapter 2: The Science Behind Intermittent Fasting

Before we move on to the topic of how intermittent fasting works, you first need to understand the problems with the current diet that people follow. Once you understand that, the necessity of following intermittent fasting will become clearer to everyone.

Why Is the Modern Diet Not Right?

Obesity is a major problem in today's world, and in the U.S alone, it is estimated that one-third of the total population is obese. Striking, isn't it? If we do the math, then the number of obese individuals amounts to a total of seventy-eight million. The problem has reached this devastating range only because it has been taken lightly and now obesity brings a whole lot of other critical problems along with it like cardiovascular disease and diabetes being the two most common ones. When you are obese, you automatically run the risk of having a stroke. Moreover, there is another fact that I'm sure is going to shock you and that is the major cause of preventable death that happens every year in America is obesity.

Now, the root of all these problems can be traced back to how our diets have drastically changed over the decades. People have turned to foods that are deep-fried and processed, and the amount of food consumption per meal has also seen a great increase. The statistics show that the total number of calories that people consume on a daily basis has increased by 400. All of this has been made possible and easier because people can easily get their hands on junk food at any nearby store at very affordable prices. And, people have simply turned a blind eye to all the bad effects of this kind of diet.

The statistics over the past decades also show that the consumption of sugar has increased in people. Today, an average person takes twenty-two teaspoons of sugar every day. When this figure is compared to your calorie intake in an entire day, it amounts to twenty-five percent of it. In the past, this figure was twenty percent less than what it is today. Now, if you think that people consume this amount of sugar directly, then you are wrong. The sugar is present in desserts, juices, and even in sauces. Sometimes, parents do not know how they are handing their kids foods that have hidden sugar content. Another thing that adds to the consumption of sugar is the soda drinks.

It was in the year 2002 when the soda drinks had started gaining popularity. Sometimes, people think that replacing soda drinks with fruit juices will do the drink, but that is just a false impression. What you have to do is reduce your overall sugar intake.

People have also increased their intake of trans fats in the form of margarine, chocolate, pastries, pizza, cereals, ice cream, fried chicken, cookies, burgers, and the list goes on and on. In recent years, people have understood and have started regulating the intake of trans fats but there are still a lot of changes that have to be made. The biggest barrier that is yet to overcome is stopping the consumption of processed fast food. No one tries to make a good and healthy breakfast when they can easily grab a pastry, donut or burger on their way to work. If you think that grabbing that packet of chips from the gas station will not do you harm then you need to rethink because it contains trans fats.

What Happens When You Fast?

Now, this is the major question that almost everyone has when they start fasting. Since we are about to begin a very important part of this book, let me clear out one major myth once and for all. Intermittent fasting is not in any way related to starving. You will often find people engaging in casual conversations and using these two words together. But this is wrong because starving is when you are not receiving the right nutrients and thus become malnourished. It has been mentioned in the Encyclopedia of Human Nutrition by Benjamin Caballero that a normal person can last for about sixty to seventy days because of his/her fat stores, and after that, they will perish. So, in short, even if you decide to do a full day fast, you are not starving yourself. All you have to make sure is that when you are in the eating window, you eat healthily and maintain proper intake of nutrients so that you do not suffer from malnutrition.

The main aim of this section is to provide you an insight into the biochemical changes that occur in your body when you fast. By the end of this chapter, you will realize how beneficial even a short fast can prove to be for your body and overall health.

Formation of Ketone Bodies

Now, if you are in the fasting window, it does not mean that your body lacks energy or something like that. Just do some background reading, and you will gain knowledge on how intermittent fasting can actually help to increase your energy levels just after the few initial weeks. And the basic reason behind this is the process of ketogenesis.

The process of ketogenesis in the body of human beings is sparked by the hormone glucagon. When the level of sugar in your blood is low (due to fasting), lipolysis starts where fatty acids are formed, and they, in turn, act as the source of energy for your body in the fasting stage. Some of the fatty acids also form ketone bodies by the process of oxidation.

If you are wondering what ketone bodies really are then here is a small explanation – when the levels of glucose in the blood are really low, that is when fatty acids get converted into ketone bodies. In our body, ketone bodies are being produced at all times, even if it is in small amounts. But in general cases, these ketone bodies will not go into your bloodstream. Instead, they undergo a process of metabolism in the liver. When you are in your eating window, then your body has glucose to turn to when it needs energy. But when you are fasting, that is when the need for an alternative energy source rises and ketone bodies jump into the scene. At that time, there is a mass production of ketone bodies as well.

There are three significant types of ketone bodies, and they are – beta-hydroxybutyrate, acetoacetate, and acetone. The first two have to be understood very well if you want to understand the science behind intermittent fasting. One of the special features of these ketone bodies is that they have the ability to cross the blood-brain barrier and they can be taken to every corner of your body through the bloodstream. The production of ketone bodies in your body will go to its peak stage after the first couple of days of fasting. But when the levels of blood ketone are considered, there you will see a rise for about 7 to 10 days starting from the day you had begun the fast. This is also the reason why intermittent fasting raises your energy levels after the first few weeks. By that time, your body becomes used to the situation where it utilizes ketone bodies as an alternative to glucose as a source of energy.

Moreover, you will often find people who claim that they feel more energized on performing intermittent fasting as compared to eating three full meals every day. Do you know the reason behind this? Well, when you eat a very heavy meal or if you keep taking such meals throughout the day, then your body is forced to remain in a state of digestion almost every hour and this takes up a lot of energy of your body. So, your body tries to stay engaged at all times and brings you fatigue.

Ghrelin

As you have read in the first chapter, one of the foremost benefits of intermittent fasting is that it is very helpful in reducing inflammation in your body. There are so many chronic diseases whose major cause is inflammation, and now, with the help of intermittent fasting, you can prevent it. When there is internal inflammation, one of the first things that will happen is that you will feel swollen and hot and when you are able to reduce your internal inflammation, you will also be able to reduce your waist size.

Now, there is a hormone called ghrelin, and it is also very popularly known as the 'hunger hormone.' It is said that ghrelin can actually help you to reduce inflammation when you are performing a fast. When you are doing intermittent fasting, the levels of ghrelin in your body increases. People who are naturally leaner have higher levels of ghrelin.

The occurrence of inflammation in your body can actually push you into a vicious cycle where you gain weight, and so, if you are serious about losing weight, then working on reducing internal inflammation is something that you should really concentrate on. People who have inflammatory diseases have been known to take the help of ghrelin but if you are fasting, then the levels of ghrelin will automatically rise in your body thus becoming a natural booster for your health.

Leptin

Now, we are going to talk about another hormone, which is very important behind the entire process that goes on during intermittent fasting. When people are performing intermittent fasting, the amount of leptin in their blood starts reducing. This particular hormone is produced in the adipose cells of your body. Their mechanism is all about inhibiting hunger. So, when the amount of leptin reduces and ghrelin increases, it is actually a response of your body towards not eating and this is also the reason why fat starts becoming the new source of energy for your body.

I know what you might be thinking that being hungry all the time is uncomfortable, but trust me when I say this, you will quickly become adapted to the entire condition. When intermittent fasting becomes your new regular routine, you will have more energy than you need and intense hunger will no longer bother you. People become so much adapted to the fact that they have food within their reach all the time that they start feeling hungry even when their body does not need food. All you have to do is break this cycle and everything will start falling in place after the first couple of weeks.

Stages of Intermittent Fasting

There is a cascade of events that are happening in your body during intermittent fasting, and all of the things that are happening during these events leave a profound effect on your overall health. In general, when you are not eating any food, the levels of glucagon rise and insulin drops which, in turn, help in the restoration of insulin sensitivity and also show improvement in the conditions of prediabetes, type 2 diabetes, and PCOS.

Six to Twelve Hours of Fasting

This phase of fasting is the post-absorptive stage when there is a reduction in the levels of glucose because all the food that you had previously eaten has been metabolized. Now, due to this, the secretion of insulin is no longer at the same level, and there is a subsequent rise in the amount of glucagon in the blood. These two events work together to signal your body that it is time to utilize glycogen (stored glucose) as an alternative form of energy. In general, an average adult is known to have stored glucose amounting to 2000 calories and with this, you can maintain the normal level of blood glucose for pretty much 24 hours.

Also, the high amount of glucagon in blood coupled with a low amount of insulin can also trigger your kidneys to excrete more amount of minerals and water. This entire process leads to glycogen being metabolized. So, when you are in this stage, you will notice that you have frequent urination, and you will be losing weight, water, and electrolytes. That is exactly why it is so essential to keep yourself properly hydrated when you are performing intermittent fasting. You also need to maintain a proper intake of electrolytes to cope with the amount that is lost.

Once you are past the six-hour fasting window, the first effect will be on your digestive system, which will start to slow down. During this fast, it gets to restore its energy and take some rest. The entire process also helps in strengthening the lining of the gut barrier and also promotes the microbiome population in the gut.

Whole Day Fasting – 24 Hours

Once you have completed a fast spanning over twenty-four hours, your body will not be able to maintain the usual level of glucose in the blood because, by this time, the entire storage of glycogen will be used. So, as an alternative measure, the body starts the production of glucose from precursors like glycerol and amino acids, that is, compounds that are non-carbohydrate in nature. The process by which this is done is termed as gluconeogenesis. If you translate the term, then the meaning stands to be the production of new glucose.

There are some people who start worrying about whether they will lose muscles because of the process of gluconeogenesis, but you don't have to worry. There is no muscle loss involved. Your body has several types of storage tissues to utilize and so isn't it a bit stupid for the body to jump to the muscles straightaway for the production of glucose? When you are fully fed, your body really works hard to gather resources so that when there is a state of low food availability, your body can utilize the stored reserve to produce energy.

Moreover, when you are fasting, it has been noticed that there is a rise in the levels of HGH or Human Growth Hormone. It is responsible for keeping the lean mass of the body intact. Once you are already twenty-four hours into the process of fasting, there is a process that takes place known as autophagy. The amino acids of your body are then sourced with the help of this process.

The process of autophagy is quite natural, and your body's way of getting rid of all the worn-out cells. It is very similar to recycling and self-cleaning. All the junky and degraded cells present in your body are killed by the cells and then new cells are generated.

One of the core processes involved in intermittent fasting is autophagy, and it is because of autophagy that intermittent fasting has gained such momentum. All the anti-aging benefits associated with intermittent fasting are possible because of the process of autophagy.

Forty-Eight Hours Fasting

Now, the energy required for your body to remain active cannot be derived from gluconeogenesis alone. That is why your body eventually moves into the state of ketosis. This is the actual fat-burning mode of the body. This stage is sometimes also known as fat adaptation because, in this stage, the main energy source of the body becomes fat and not glucose.

Fatty acids and glycerol are formed by the process of metabolism of stored fat. The fatty acids so formed are utilized by various tissues in the body but the only exception is the brain because it can only use ketone and glucose and nothing else. On the other hand, glycerol is utilized to maintain a stable blood glucose concentration.

But your brain always has a high demand for energy, and when the amount of glucose is not present in the required amounts, the formation of ketone bodies starts. Ketone bodies, on the other hand, are very efficient molecules that serve as an alternative source of fuel in time of need and also promote the brain-derived neurotrophic factor production or BDNF. Now, you might be wondering what the function of this particular factor is. Well, they help in the repair and growth of brain cells and also shield them against any amount of cellular stress. This, in turn, elevates mental clarity and helps you to focus well.

Seventy-Two Hours Fasting

When you have been fasting for about 72 hours, then the levels of insulin in your blood are at its lowest. Another thing that happens is that your body has totally adapted to deriving energy from fat. Ketone bodies and fat molecules have become the major sources of energy for your body. Also, to preserve the amount of lean mass in your body, the amount of HGH is also high.

By the time you are fasting for three days, autophagy is going on in full motion, and a direct result of this is that your immune system is fixed and rejuvenated. Over time, the cells of your immune system also undergo degradation and so, autophagy triggers the formation of new cells in your immune system.

So, now you might have understood how fasting is more like a lifestyle choice, and it comes with several benefits. When you understand what goes on at the physiological level during intermittent fasting, it will be an added boost for you to go on fasting and reap its benefits. But yes, it is also true that if you are a beginner, you should not jump into doing a 72-hour fast. Start small and then work your way up the ladder.

What Is Autophagy?

The origin of the word 'autophagy' is Greek. Now, there are always certain types of machinery inside your cell that are worn out, and if the body keeps maintaining them, then that will be an immense waste of energy that the body cannot afford to do. Hence, the decision is to get rid of them and the process followed is termed as autophagy. It is a very regulated and orderly method of recycling old cells. The process was discovered for the first time in the year 1962. The term was decided by Christian de Duve who later on won a Nobel prize. When the damaged parts of proteins are marked for elimination from the cell, it is the task of the lysosome to complete the task. There is a kinase by the name of mTOR and this kinase acts as the most important regulator of the process of autophagy. The process is promoted when the kinase is dormant but the moment it becomes active, there is a suppression of autophagy in the cells.

Now, let's move on to the next thing that you need to understand in this respect, and that is – how is autophagy activated? Well, to put it simply, whenever you are in the fasting mode for a certain period of time, autophagy gets activated. Also, when fasting is triggering autophagy, it is also triggering something else at the same time and that is the production of the growth hormone. So, when autophagy is eliminating all the worn-out cells, the human growth hormone leads to the replacement of those old cells by new ones. Thus, this is how renovation happens.

But you also need to understand that autophagy does not simply happen like that. There are a lot of factors that control and regulate it. This is because if autophagy was not kept under control, it could easily have negative effects and destroy your overall health. When all these junks and old proteins are not eliminated, and they start accumulating in your body, the first thing that happens is that you suffer from neurodegenerative problems like Parkinson's or Alzheimer's diseases (AD). There is either amyloid beta protein or Tau protein that accumulates in your brain when you suffer from AD. Thus, the entire system gets clogged and cannot function the way it should to stay healthy. But if the process of autophagy were to perform as it should, there would be no junk proteins in the first place and so people would not have to suffer from conditions like AD.

The process of autophagy also has to stop at a certain time, and that is caused by eating. Yes, you might be surprised but eating is the way to stop autophagy. In simpler words, when you break the fast, you are stopping autophagy. Several proteins, glucose, and insulin together stop autophagy and you do not really require huge amounts. Even a small amount of insulin can instantly stop the process of autophagy. Now, if you are thinking that you can make your body perform autophagy simply by limiting calories, then you are wrong. It does not happen that way. It only happens when you perform a proper fast.

But you also need to ensure that there is a balance. You cannot let autophagy to go on endlessly. In the same way, if there is a very little amount of autophagy, then too it is of no use. So, what you have to do is maintain a proper balance between fasting and feasting, and only then can you ensure proper cleansing at a cellular level.

Will Autophagy Help in Boosting Your Overall Health?

The simple answer would be yes. But then you definitely have to perform intermittent fasting under proper guidance and maintain a balance for autophagy to be truly helpful for your health. If you overdo the process, then it will be detrimental and not helpful. Almost everyone I know would say that they want their life to be long and happy and honestly, who would say no to such a thing, right? And do you know what the best part is? Autophagy can actually help you live longer. The best way to ensure that your body goes into the state of autophagy is to engage in intermittent fasting. It is a very easy process to follow if you are just a beginner.

The statistics all over the world will show you how obesity is becoming a major source of concern for everyone and what a great impact it has on your health. And the worst part about all of this is that obesity is not any singular problems. It has a lot of baggage with it because of which you will face severe complications. The very foremost of complications are those of heart and also diabetes. You can even get gout and stroke. The list is quite long, and I don't want to scare you with it. What I believe in is prevention especially when it is entirely in your own hands. If you are careful now and perform intermittent fasting then you will be able to keep your Body Mass Index is a healthy range and steer clear of such nasty problems.

Limiting the number of calories you consume in a particular day and also causing a gradual reduction of portion sizes is something you can start with. You will also get a diet plan at the end of this book, which will make the planning part easier. And once you get the hang of it, varying the plan with recipes of your own will become easier too. Moreover, fasting is an excellent way of limiting calorie intake without even worrying much about it. Also, you are literally guiding your body towards autophagy and so it starts the process of self-cleansing.

One of the major benefits of autophagy is that you can keep neurodegenerative disorders at bay like Parkinson's and Alzheimer's and even dementia. Also, newer and newer proteins and cells are created, and your lifespan increases because your body no longer has to function with the old and worn-out cells. And last but not least, if your main goal is to lose weight, then too intermittent fasting and autophagy can help you do so by bringing your BMI in a healthier range.

Chapter 3: How Does I. F. Help in Weight Loss?

Now that you have a basic idea about things, it is time that we dive deeper into the science behind intermittent fasting and really look into how everything goes on behind the scenes.

What Is the Mechanism Behind Losing Weight?

If you truly want to understand how you can lose weight or what makes you gain weight, then understanding certain hormonal functions is also important. This, in turn, will also help you understand the working mechanism of intermittent fasting. Now, there are two very important hormones in your body that control the levels of blood glucose, and these are – insulin and glucagon. And there is another pair about whom you must have some knowledge and they are brown fat and white fat. You will keep gaining and losing weight and it is quite a natural fluctuation that the human body goes through. In order to understand this process, having full knowledge of these pairs is essential.

Insulin and Glucagon

You might have already done some research on how insulin is related to your blood glucose or blood sugar levels. But what we are going to discuss here is how any of this is related to gaining weight. Now, the place where insulin is made in your body is none other than the pancreas, and this insulin, in turn, is responsible for maintaining proper levels of blood glucose.

People suffer from hyperglycemia when the levels of glucose in their blood become high. Similarly, they suffer from hypoglycemia when the levels of glucose in their blood become low. When you are eating food, there is a subsequent rise in the levels of glucose in your blood. This is because the food is being digested as a result of which glucose is formed by the transformation of carbohydrates. This glucose is then utilized by the organ systems so that they can get the energy to perform their activities. Now, when you think about carbs, I bet that the first food items that come to your mind are probably something along the lines of pasta and bread, but there are so many veggies and fruits that are rich in carbs as well.

Now, when there is a rise in the levels of glucose in the blood, insulin is released from the pancreas. The task of insulin is to signal the fats, muscles, and liver in your body to start the absorption of glucose from the bloodstream. This is the actual process in which the different organ systems derive energy. When the amount of glucose is more in the blood than what is actually required, the glucose gets stored in the form of glycogen in the liver. Sometimes, insulin helps in converting excess glucose into fatty acids. The adipose tissues in your body are where the fats are stored.

Now, there are three things that are inhibited by the presence of insulin, and they are as follows – gluconeogenesis, glycogenolysis, and lipolysis. So, lipolysis is when your body engages in the breakdown of fats in order to derive energy for day-to-day activities. Glycogenolysis is when usable glucose is formed by the breakdown of glycogen. The process is inhibited by the presence of insulin. And lastly, gluconeogenesis is when the non-carbohydrate sources act as the substrate from which glucose is created.

So, we have two hormones working behind the scenes. The three mechanisms mentioned above are set into motion by the presence of glucagon, and these mechanisms are the reason why there is a rise in the levels of glucose in your blood. But the presence of insulin has the capability of inhibiting these mechanisms and then reducing the levels of glucose in the blood.

What Are the Barriers That Women Face When It Comes to Weight Loss?

There was a study that was conducted by the Yale Journal of Biology and Medicine, and in it, it was stated how women are more prone to being obese than men. In fact, the chances of a woman being obese are twice that of a man. Now, if you are wondering why then here are the reasons –

Hormones

One of the biggest reasons for women being more prone to weight gain is their hormonal makeup. Factors like diet, aging, and stress play a big role in the alteration of hormones like estrogen, cortisol, and progesterone, and obesity is a by-product of all these changes taken together. The reason behind women not being adapted to these hormonal changes is because our diets are being increasingly composed of foods that are highly processed.

Also, the process of storing fat in the body of a woman is influenced by the hormone estrogen, which is also known as the female sex hormone. One of the most common signs of aging in women is that they start gaining weight and losing muscles and the major reason is the reduction in the level of estrogen. An important event in the life of women over the age of 50 is menopause and with menopause comes the reduction of estrogen in the body.

Metabolism

The process of metabolism that is present in women is not the same as that in men, and there are some differences that will show you how it acts as a barrier in weight loss. The amount of lean muscles is more in men than in women and this greater number of lean muscles is one of the reasons why the resting metabolic rate of men is higher. There is a scientific reason behind it too. The efficiency of muscles to burn calories is much more than fats. So, possessing a greater number of lean muscles automatically means that they are going to burn more calories. So, even if a man is not performing any strenuous physical activity, he will be burning more calories than a woman doing the same thing.

The process becomes worse because of the fact that the storage of fat is also different between the two genders. The fat, in the case of women, is mostly stored in areas like thighs, buttocks, and hips. And any fitness expert can confirm this that these are exactly the regions which need a lot of effort to shed fat from.

Emotions

Yes, no matter how you feel about this one but emotions do play a big role when it comes to weight loss, especially in women. The American Journal of Clinical Nutrition confirms the fact that emotional eating is something that women are more engaging with than men. It was in the year 2013 that this study was published. Some of the findings that this research had are as follows –

- Women are more inclined towards maintaining a diet, but maintaining something consistently for a period of time also requires an immense amount of motivation and willpower. Both these factors can be adversely affected by fluctuation in emotions that can, in turn, lead to stress. Also, it was found that emotional eating was a case that was more common in those women who were following some kind of diet and not that much common in those who were not following any diet at all. Thus, women need to be more aware of the factors that can cause stress and trigger an emotional eating response.
- Probably the worst part about someone engaging in emotional eating is that they will not go for a healthy smoothie or kale salad in case something is bothering them, or they are utterly depressed. Instead, they will reach out for sugary stuff like ice cream, cookies, and chocolates, all of whom have a lot of calories.
- Lastly, it is not that much to break out of a pattern of emotional eating. But at the end of the day, emotional eating is nothing but a learned behavior, and such behaviors can be unlearnt with proper effort and willpower. But you have to realize that you are in this vicious cycle and you have to break free otherwise if you go too deep into it, then breaking free will become equally difficult.

Genetics

The genetic makeup of a person is also one of the reasons why they are more prone to obesity than others. For example, if every woman in your lineage had a tendency to be over the average BMI, then there are high chances that you will have the same tendency too. So, no matter how much effort you put into weight loss, these factors will still be working against you.

So, the only thing that you have to do is keep reminding yourself not to expect any results soon. In order to lower your BMI, one of the key steps to take is to live an incremental lifestyle. But yes, intermittent fasting definitely is an effective tool to help you in your weight loss journey.

Relation Between Weight Loss and Intermittent Fasting

Now that we are talking so much about fat and glucose and the difference between them as a source of energy, you must have understood that even fat is nothing but the body's way of storing energy. In order to make fat more easily available to your body, there are certain changes taking place in your body during the fasting window. These are all related to the metabolism of the body, and they are explained below –

- **Insulin Levels** – The level of insulin in the human body shows an increase whenever you are eating something. In the same manner, the opposite happens when you do not eat food; that is, the level of insulin decreases. And when this happens, the process of fat burning is facilitated.
- **Human Growth Hormone or HGH** – The levels of this hormone increase to five or six times its usual amount during the fasting window. The main functions of this hormone include loss of fat and gain in muscles, but apart from this, it helps in a lot of other things as well.
- **Norepinephrine** – The fat cells receive norepinephrine when you are on a fast as a message sent by the nervous system. After this, the formation of fatty acids takes place in the body. Then, they serve as an alternative source of fuel to cater to your body's energy requirements.

A fasting period of about forty-eight hours can really boost your body's metabolic rate by as much as 3.6-14%, and this was published in The American Journal of Physiology. But similarly, if you do not want your metabolic rates to go off the rails and show drastic reduction instead, then you need to keep fasting periods under control.

The process of weight loss happens merely through a deficit of calories, and that is exactly what happens when you engage in intermittent fasting. Since you are skipping meals, you are reducing your calorie intake. This does not depend on the method of intermittent fasting you are following. No matter what method you follow, you will still be reducing your calories. But there is also something else to keep in mind here. When you are in your eating window, you have to limit your calorie consumption and not overdo it because if you eat too much, there will no longer be any calorie deficit and your fasting will not bring any results.

The ways in which intermittent fasting helps your body to lose weight are as follows –

- **Reduction in Stored Fat** – During the fasting window, both the amounts of glucose and glycogen are depleted so fast, and so insulin sensitivity improves after a certain period of time. This means that your body gradually becomes used to utilizing lower insulin amounts as a result of a reduced blood sugar level. Also, the efficiency of utilization of glucose also improves. Moreover, since the amount of insulin present in your blood in the fasting period is limited, the blood sugar is also not able to reach any other areas than where it is supposed so. So, it does not get added to the fat storage of your body. Thus, the amount of fat that you have already lost will not be regained.

- **Better Muscle Growth** – As I have already mentioned earlier, during the intermittent fasting, there is an increase in the HGH levels. An increase in HGH alone would not have created much of an impact, but in the case of intermittent fasting, not only is there a rise in the level of HGH, but calorie restriction is also practiced. Both of these factors together can do wonders to help in fat loss. There is a process of metabolism that is set into motion by HGH and for that, the fat stored in your body is utilized.

- **Increase in Lean Muscles** – In most of the weight loss strategies that are there, one of the major drawbacks is that almost all of them, in some or the other way, lead to the reduction of lean muscles. But intermittent fasting is really an exception to this and does not cause any reduction in muscles. The direct result of a decrease in muscle mass is that your body's requirement of calories is also reduced. This means that no matter how much you restrict your calories, there is always a surplus that is created. So, intermittent fasting ensures that none of this happens. In fact, with this procedure, you can not only lose weight but also maintain a nice figure with proper lean muscle mass.

- **Lesser Cravings** – Food cravings are definitely one of the biggest barriers that lead to unsuccessful diet plans, and the same happens for intermittent fasting too. But there is also a plus point here. After the first couple of weeks, as the insulin sensitivity starts to improve with intermittent fasting, so does the occurrence of these cravings. The more you practice intermittent fasting, the more tolerant you will become towards hunger. Moreover, satiety levels will increase and that is also one of the reasons why people experience a lesser amount of cravings.

The visceral area of the woman's body is the part where all the fat accumulates, but with the help of intermittent fasting, you can reduce that fat. Also, visceral fat becomes a high-risk factor for chronic diseases like colorectal cancer, type 2 diabetes and also cardiovascular diseases. Moreover, the chances of your arteries getting blocked increases when the amount of visceral fat in your body is high. But in the case of intermittent fasting, there is a reduction of not only subcutaneous fat but also visceral fat. And since autophagy is promoted when you fast, there is an added advantage. Autophagy inhibits the formation of any new visceral fat.

Chapter 4: What Foods Should You Include?

Fasting is something whose presence is found throughout history. Whether it was used as a spiritual tool or for expressing political dissent, fasting was present in all eras. Because of the immense anti-aging and weight loss benefits, intermittent fasting has gained a lot of traction in recent years. But what you eat during your eating window also matters to realize the benefits of the process. So, here are some of the food items that you should eat when you are performing intermittent fasting.

Water

Water is the most important thing to have when you are fasting. Intermittent fasting does not bar you from drinking water even when you are fasting. In fact, if you want to prevent your body from getting dehydrated, water is something that you should have. It is not recommended for any human being to go for such a long stretch of time without any fluids. Almost every process that goes on inside your body requires water. Moreover, when you drink water at regular intervals, it can even help you keep the hunger in check. When the glycogen is burned to get energy, there is an immense amount of shortage of electrolytes and fluid in your body, and to replace that, you need to drink water. You should drink at least eight glasses of water every day. This will keep dehydration at bay and also ensure that there is proper blood flow. Moreover, you will have proper joint health, and your muscles will also remain in good condition.

Coffee

When you are performing intermittent fasting, you will have to skip meals and that is no secret. But the first question that comes to everyone's minds is that what about coffee? It is said that when you consume very low or zero-calorie beverages, then you are not harming your intermittent fasting regime in any way. And coffee falls in that category. There are about three calories in a cup of black coffee, which is approximately 240 ml. There are some trace minerals and very small amounts of proteins as well. In short, the nutrients that are present in black coffee will not break your fast or cause any type of significant metabolic change. Some people who have been performing intermittent fasting have also said that black coffee really helped them stick to their fast and not give up midway. This is because, in some ways, coffee can help to suppress your appetite. But you definitely have to ensure that the coffee is black and that you are not adding either sugar or milk.

Moreover, coffee has certain metabolic effects of its own that can actually boost fasting. As you must have already learned that there are several chronic illnesses whose root cause is inflammation. But research was published, which showed that when coffee and intermittent fasting are combined together, it can actually help in the reduction of inflammation inside the body. There have also been studies that show that the risk to type-2-diabetes can be reduced by the consumption of coffee. In short, the benefits of coffee and intermittent fasting are the same in several respects and there is no harm in having black coffee during the fasting periods.

Grains That Are Minimally Processed

All this talk about having a low-carb diet does not necessarily mean that carbs are your enemy. Whole foods can provide you a lot of energy and are also digested easily. So, you have to include them in your diet but do it in a strategical manner so that you don't end up consuming too many carbs. Moreover, foods like whole oats are highly rich in antioxidants, which are important for your body. This not only helps in reducing your high levels of blood pressure but also protects you from colon cancer. Moreover, they contain special compounds known as beta-glucans. These compounds are nothing but soluble fibers that help in the absorption of other nutrients. You should also consider including buckwheat in your diet because it is rich in so many different nutrients like B vitamins, iron, magnesium, manganese, phosphorus, and copper. Moreover, they are gluten-free naturally.

Lentils

If you do not know this, then you must know that there are so many health benefits associated with lentils and so they are advised to be included in the diet of a person performing intermittent fasting. Firstly, I would like to mention that lentils are rich in a special compound known as polyphenols. These compounds are quite active, and they help your body to fight against so many things including cancer, heart diseases, and also UV rays. Moreover, just a cup of cooked lentils can give you as much as eighteen grams of protein. They are also a very good source of iron and this particular mineral is important to ensure that you have a proper flow of blood in your body. The lentils are also a good source of fiber. So, if you are performing intermittent fasting to lose weight, then lentils are a must. For women who are above the age of 50, lentils help to strengthen your bones by giving you a boost of calcium. Menopause brings troubles with sleeping and lentils can help you with that too because they provide your body with magnesium. A cup of cooked lentils contains 71 mg of magnesium.

Raspberries

Raspberries are also advised to a person who is following intermittent fasting. You might really be surprised by the endless list of benefits that raspberries have. They are packed with nutrients. Just like every other vitamin and mineral, your body needs Vitamin C to ensure that the immune system is working properly. A cup of raspberries can fulfill more than half of your daily target of vitamin C. They also contain Vitamin K and manganese, and both of these are important for supporting good bone health.

Another good thing about raspberries is that their sugar content is really low. In each cup of raspberries, there are only five grams of sugar, whereas one medium-sized apple will give you twenty grams of sugar. So, when you are trying to lose weight and yet you need to eat fruits, raspberries can be a great option. Raspberries are also one of the best sources of antioxidants. Thus, they help you control obesity, cardiovascular problems, and even diabetes. One of the main causes of premature aging is the occurrence of internal inflammation and the antioxidants of raspberries help to reduce inflammation. Moreover, they also have compounds that help in the process of DNA repair.

You will get approximately eight grams of fiber from a cup of raspberries, and so they have a high level of satiety. When you are performing intermittent fasting, you need to eat foods that are low in carbs but also high in fiber so that you do not feel hungry often. The fiber content also helps in keeping your digestive system in good condition.

Seitan

For those who want to avoid animal-based proteins, seitan is the best alternative. This particular animal-protein substitute has life-extending properties and is really good for women above the age of 50. Moreover, you do not have to take any hassle in cooking seitan. It can be cooked very easily and in the blink of an eye. You can bake it by slicing into pieces, just like meat. It can also be deep-fried or you can enjoy it by slathering it in barbeque sauce and then having it as a main dish with some salad at the sides. Or, if you are in the mood for a lighter flavor, then you can steam the seitan or make a hearty winter stew.

Hummus

If we are talking about plant-based proteins, then hummus is equally nutritious. You will get only 166 calories from 100 grams of hummus. The protein content is 7.9 grams in each serving. As I have already mentioned before, one of the biggest things to fight in the old age is the internal inflammation that happens in your body and leads to several chronic diseases. Hummus is rich in antioxidants, which, in turn, have some amazing anti-inflammatory benefits. They are also a rich source of dietary fiber and you get approximately six grams of dietary fiber in every serving of hummus. So, if you are someone who suffers from constipation, the consumption of hummus will soften your stools and help them to pass through easily. They also help in maintaining the good health of your colon.

Because of the low glycemic index value of hummus, they help in keeping blood sugar levels under control. It also contains ingredients that are heart-healthy, for example, olive oil. The several properties of hummus also help in bringing your BMI in a healthy range. The levels of ghrelin are also reduced and so you won't feel those hunger pangs during fasting. If you have sandwiches, then you can easily have hummus in place of mayonnaise. But in case you think you want to make your own hummus, then the two most important ingredients you need are tahini and garlic.

Salmon

One of the common food items that you will find in every intermittent fasting diet is salmon. This is because it reduces several risk factors associated with old age and is also full of nutrients. For starters, they are rich in omega-3-fatty acids. They will not only help you in decreasing inflammation, reduce cancer, reduce levels of blood pressure, and also improve the health of the arteries. Moreover, salmon are an incredible source of protein. They help in maintaining proper bone health and also does not let anything happen to your muscle mass even when you are losing weight. Moreover, during the aging process, there may be chances of losing weight, which is reduced by the consumption of salmon.

Another importance of salmon is that they are a great source of B-vitamins. Potassium is another mineral that is present in high amounts in salmon. If you do not know this, then potassium helps in maintaining proper levels of blood pressure, and thus, you can steer clear of risks of stroke. Lastly, salmon is rich in an important trace mineral – selenium. It helps in decreasing antibodies of thyroid especially in those who suffer from autoimmune diseases of the thyroid and also helps in the improvement of bone health.

Blueberries

Blueberries might be small, but don't let their size fool you into thinking that they do not have any benefits. They are packed of all good things even though their size is small. Another great thing about them is that they are sweet and have a great taste and yet so much nutritious. Being rich in antioxidants, blueberries can help your body to scavenge all the free radicals that are quite harmful and can lead to several chronic problems and neurodegenerative disorders. The flavonoids are the major antioxidants present in the blueberries. Your DNA undergoes oxidative damage almost every day and it is truly unavoidable. This damage increases even more with advancing age. But blueberries can prevent this damage because of their antioxidant content.

Moreover, when the LDL cholesterol levels in your body are oxidized, it leads to several heart problems, all of which can be prevented by the consumption of blueberries. In short, blueberries can be your best friend when it comes to maintaining heart health. These fruits have also been known to lower your levels of blood pressure. When there is oxidative stress in your body, one of the major organs to be affected is your brain, and this is also a part of the aging process. But the intake of blueberries can maintain healthy neurons in the brain thus causing significant improvements in the process of cell signaling.

Blueberries are also rich in anthocyanins, which help in improving insulin resistance and thus also help in keeping blood sugar within healthy limits. With an improvement in insulin sensitivity, the direct result is that you will have lesser chances of developing type 2 diabetes.

Chapter 5: Some Practical Tips to Start Intermittent Fasting

The most delicate phase of intermittent fasting is the time when you just start it. That is the time when most people give up on it. If people indeed lose some weight, then they get so excited that they start falling back to their old and unhealthy lifestyles and if they do not get the results they wished for, they too they think that intermittent fasting is a complete waste of time. If you have been doing it for a week and got some results, it is really great and I totally appreciate but in order to reap the full benefits, you need to keep practicing it and make it a lifestyle habit. So, here are some tips that will help you start intermittent fasting the right way.

Break Your Fast With the Right Foods

At the end of a fast, when you eat something after a long time, eating the wrong foods can actually spike up the levels of blood sugar, and so you need to be careful about what you are eating. The same thing happens with the level of insulin in the body because they are never consistent. But intermittent fasting has profound benefits when it comes to lowering the levels of insulin in the body. When there is an elevation in the levels of insulin, that is exactly when the body stops burning fat.

Similarly, if insulin is present in huge quantities in your bloodstream, then it will be highly difficult for your body to burn any fat. Now one of the main aims of engaging in intermittent fasting is so that your body can go into a fat-burning mode. So suppose you have complete an almost perfect fast, but in the end, you break it by consuming the wrong type of food, then all that effort that went into the fast was for nothing and the insulin levels will also start to spike.

So, in order to support the process of fat burning, you need to choose foods that are wholesome, and they should not be processed foods. The insulin levels are very heavily impacted when you consume carbs, so your goal is to stick to foods that are low in carbs. Protein has only a moderate impact but there are certain dairy products that can leave quite the impact. The least amount of impact is left by fats and that is also why the keto diet is encouraged when you are on an intermittent fasting regime.

So, stop indulging in carbs or dairy when you are breaking your fast. Sometimes, people overdo it when they break the fast because they think that they somehow have to compensate for the fasting. But it is not that. Also, you need to remember that you can get carried away easily if you are not focused enough. So, when you eat, limit your calories and stick to the food items that have been mentioned in the previous chapter.

Fast for Longer Periods Once You Are Accustomed to the Process

Whenever you fast, the amount of insulin in the blood is lowered. So, that is when the body starts burning fat. Thus, the longer you can fast, the longer you can allow your body to stay in the fat-burning mode. But you should not jump into long fasts right in the beginning. At first, you have to master the protocols mentioned in the short term fasts, and then you have to move on to the longer ones. Extended hours of fasting can be an entire day or you can also try out the 48-hour fast once the full day fasting becomes easy.

The advice that I give to every beginner is that you should start with the 16/8 method because in this, you will have to fast for a period of sixteen hours, and if you decide to skip breakfast, then more than half the fasting window is spent sleeping. So, the process becomes quite easier. After you have performed the 16/8 method for about a week or so and you are feeling that it is becoming easy for you, start by doing a 20-hour fast daily. This means that the eating window becomes really short and you have to squeeze it to four hours. Even if the timeframe is short, you can have two small meals here.

Once you have mastered this too, then you can practice the Warrior Diet, which was mentioned at the beginning of this book. In simpler words, you will have only one meal every day. When you have reached the expert level, then you can take your fasts to 36 hours or 48 hours. At first, such long fasting periods will seem impossible and that is perfectly normal. You are not supposed to do it once but you have to work your way up there. The more you fast consistently, you will notice that the feeling of hunger has started to become blunt. When you are fasting for longer periods, the limitation on calories is increased and fat burning increases too.

Steer Clear of Artificial Drinks

When people are fasting, especially beginners, have this tendency to reach out for the artificial drinks in the form of diet soda, energy drinks, flavored beverages, or even juices. They think that since these drinks claim to have low sugar content, they won't do any harm. But what they don't understand is that these drinks still contain a huge amount of artificial sweeteners that can harm your health.

In order to keep your body hydrated, the only liquid that you should have is water. And when you are doing intermittent fasting, there is no limitation to the amount of water you can drink. Some other drinks that are allowed during intermittent fasting are tea and black coffee, but there should be no sugar. You can also have herbal teas but the criteria remain the same – there should be no milk or sugar in them. These alternatives can easily be swapped in for a soda or other artificial drinks and you can enjoy your fasting windows.

Keep Yourself Busy

This is truly a very truthful tip because if you want your fast to be successful, then you also have to simultaneously keep yourself busy doing something or the other. It can be anything like pursuing a hobby, engaging in your favorite pastime or even work. You can do anything that will involve not thinking about food. This is one of the best ways in which you can adapt to the process of intermittent fasting. In order to be successful with the process, your task is to develop the right mentality and staying will help you with that and this will also make fasts of extended periods bearable.

If you decide to start your fast post-dinner, then that sorts out most of the problem. Do you know why? It is because the maximum portion of the time will be spent sleeping. That is why beginners are always advised to start their fast post-dinner. Now, when you are breaking your fast, if you have the meal at around noon, then it can seem quite a long stretch of time to not do anything and sit idle. This is how you will be getting the cravings. So, you need to figure out a way to fill up your mornings so that you can divert your mind from the thought of food. Do some type of productive work. When you are waiting to break your fast with a meal, the last few hours are really crucial and that is also when people lose their patience and break their fast early.

Have Proper Sleep

Whether you are into intermittent fasting or not, sleep will always be essential for you, and it is a universal truth. When you are asleep, your body works to repair your old and worn-out cells. So, sleeping properly is very crucial. You must also know that when you are sleeping, your body burns a certain amount of calories which is crucial to your weight loss journey. This also helps in giving a boost to your metabolism. The fat burning process will make your body undergo a lot of changes in the fasting window.

When you are doing a fast, sometimes you might have the tendency to overeat, and the biggest contributor to this feeling is stress. There are so many people who engage in stress eating. And the worst part about all of this is that stress eating is never related to healthy foods. The foods that stressful people reach out to are sugary in nature and full of carbs. But you have to understand something here – your stress will not be relieved if you have more carbs. Although they help in the production of serotonin which, in turn, makes people feel calmer. So, people think that carbs will help them cope with stress. But this is actually nothing more than a trap! So, to avoid this and avoid the overconsumption of carbs, you need to build a proper mindset so that you can cope with stress and keep it at bay while you are fasting.

Stay Away From Unsupportive People

When you are starting something new, it is very natural on your part to tell others about it, especially the ones you think you are close to. And then, you also seek their approval on the matter not that it is required but it will simply put your mind at ease. But in most cases, your peers or sometimes even your family members might not like the idea and they might even reject your ideas. This happens quite often. Think about all those times when you had just started a new venture and you simply couldn't stop yourself from telling it to others. But the moment you speak with someone else, they shoot you down. This can discourage you to great extents, and sometimes, the criticism they state might not even be true.

It is difficult to start something new or make certain changes in life. The same goes for intermittent fasting – it is a completely new eating plan, and sticking by it for the long-term can be hard. But once you are fully into it, you are definitely going to feel awesome. Starting is probably the hardest part of it all. You need a lot of willpower to start it and even then, you might have several doubts. Now, in this situation, if a friend or a stranger comes to you and says that your idea of fasting is completely bogus, then imagine the disappointment you would feel. The feelings can be so strong that it can make a person feel depressed.

So, sometimes, intermittent fasting is best when practiced with those who appreciate it, and if you do not have such people in your life, then practice it on your own. Never force anyone to join the journey if they are not willing to. If you usually go out with your friends for dinner, then reserve your fasting window for when you are home or you are not socializing, for example, at night and in the morning. If you do it this way, then you can skip on the process of explaining to others why you are doing what you are doing.

Follow a Ketogenic Diet

Intermittent fasting gives you enough room to practice flexibility with your diets, but the focus should be more on fats and proteins instead of carbs. You have already learned about foods to include in your diet in the previous chapter. You have to remember that ketosis is promoted by the keto diet and so if you want your body to remain in the fat-burning state for a longer period of time, then a keto diet is your best option.

Follow these tips and maintain your fast regularly. If you are not getting results right away, be patient. Don't give up midway. Everyone might not have the same response to intermittent fasting, and so you need to continue your fast without making mistakes.

Finally, let me give you this very last tip: if you are finding this book useful, your amazon review could help other people to start practicing Intermittent Fasting.

Chapter 6: Intermittent Fasting 10-Days Meal Plan

Day 1
Meal 1 – 1 pm – Summer Minestrone

Total Prep & Cooking Time: 30 minutes
Yields: Four servings
Nutrition Facts: Calories: 185 | Carbs: 29g | Protein: 7g | Fat: 6g
| Fiber: 5g

Ingredients:

A quarter cup of parmesan (grated)
One small sized carrot (thinly sliced)
One small sized zucchini (slit into pieces of half-inch each)
Eight ounces of red potatoes (slit into pieces of half-inch each)
One large-sized onion (chopped finely)
Two cloves of garlic (chopped finely)
One tablespoon of oil
Four cups of vegetable broth (low sodium)
One yellow squash (slit into pieces of half-inch each)
Half a cup of peas (frozen)
A cup of basil (fresh, chopped roughly)
To taste: Salt and Pepper
Bread crust for serving

Method:

1. Pour oil in large saucepan and heat on medium. Add onion. Sprinkle salt and pepper according to taste and cook them well, keeping the saucepan covered for about eight minutes.
2. To the mixture, add garlic and broil for a minute and add vegetable broth (low-sodium) and red potatoes; simmer for five minutes. Add carrot, yellow squash, and zucchini; simmer for three minutes.
3. After adding frozen peas, simmer for about three minutes until the veggies are tender.
4. Serve with sprinkled parmesan (grated) and fresh basil. Enjoy with crusty bread.

Meal 2 – 4 pm – Honey Almond Granola Bars

Total Prep & Cooking Time: 40 minutes
Yields: Ten servings
Nutrition Facts: Calories: 161 | Carbs: 18g | Protein: 4g | Fat: 9g
|Fiber: 3g

Ingredients:

One tsp. of cinnamon (ground)
Three tbsps. each of
- Pure honey
- Olive oil, extra virgin (substitute- coconut oil or butter)

Two cups rolled oats, old fashioned (about one hundred and seventy grams)
One tbsp. of vanilla extract
Three fourth cup of almonds, sliced (about seventy-five grams)
To taste: Sea salt

Method:

1. Set temperature of the oven to three hundred and fifty degrees Fahrenheit. Use aluminum foil to line the baking sheet.
2. Take a medium bowl to mix almonds (sliced) and oats.
3. Take a small bowl to mix cinnamon, olive oil, vanilla extract, salt, and honey and hurl with nuts and oats to coat them well.
4. Use a baking sheet, spread a layer of the mixture on it, and bake for about thirty minutes (stir every eight to ten minutes until it turns golden brown). Keep an eye to stop the granola from being over-baked.
5. Allow the granola to cool down after transferring into a cooling rack.
6. Refrigerate the extra granola for two weeks.

Meal 3 – 6 pm – Kale Chips

Total Prep & Cooking Time: 20 minutes
Yields: 6 servings
Nutrition Facts: Calories: 58| Carbs: 7.6g | Protein: 2.5g | Fat: 2.8g |Fiber:1.5g

Ingredients:

One tsp. of salt (seasoned)
One bunch of kale
One tbsp. of olive oil

Method:

1. Set temperature of the oven to one hundred and seventy-five degrees Celsius. Use a parchment paper to twine around a cookie sheet (non-insulated).
2. Remove the thick stems of kale carefully with a knife, tear into small pieces that are easy to bite. Wash the pieces thoroughly and dry them using a salad spinner.
3. Drizzle some olive oil over the kale pieces and sprinkle some amount of sea salt.
4. Bake them for fifteen minutes till edges are brown and keep an eye to check the kale pieces so that you can prevent over-burning.

Meal 4 – 9 pm – Blackberry Glazed Chicken

Total Prep & Cooking Time: 20 minutes
Yields: 4-6 servings
Nutrition Facts: Calories: 223 | Carbs: 1.1g | Protein: 35g
|Fat: 7.5g | Fiber: 0.1g

Ingredients:

For marinade,
Two tbsps. each of
- steaks seasoning
- white sugar

Desirable hot sauce (few shakes)
One cup of olive oil
Six chicken breasts (three pounds in total)
Half a cup of vinegar (balsamic)
Two cups of blackberries (mashed)

For glaze,
A quarter cup of vinegar (balsamic)
One tbsp. of cornstarch
A cup of blackberries
Half a cup each of
- white sugar
- cold water

Method:

1. Use a medium bowl to mash the blueberries and add in a Ziploc bag (large one). Add half a cup of vinegar (balsamic), two tbsps. of white sugar, hot sauce, olive oil and steak seasoning to the bag and shake it well so that all ingredients get mixed up properly.
2. Store the mixture in a fridge (the range can be from four to twenty-four hours). Twirl every two hours.
3. Heat a grill. Thick chicken breasts can be cooked evenly using a rolling pin (or meat mallet). The rolling pin will help to pound down the chicken breasts.

Preparation of glaze,

1. Use a small saucepan to mix cornstarch and cold water with a whip and put on medium heat. Add a quarter cup of balsamic vinegar, half cup of white sugar and one cup of blueberries, mash the berries. Stir for four minutes to make a thick mixture. Meanwhile, you set the oven to low heat and occasionally stir, cook the chicken.
2. Let the chicken grill for three to five minutes on one side, and the other side for four minutes. You are recommended to use a meat thermometer to keep a check on cooking the chicken.
3. Serve with warm glaze on the top and enjoy.

Day 2
Meal 1 – 1 pm – Avocado and Charred Shrimp Salad

Total Prep & Cooking Time: 25 minutes
Yields: Four servings
Nutrition Facts: Calories: 420 | Carbs: 20g | Protein: 35g
|Fat: 23.5g | Fiber: 4g

Ingredients:

Half a bunch of upland watercress
A half red onion (small and thinly sliced)
A half small pineapple, trimmed and peeled (cut into pieces of half-inch each)
Kosher salt
10.5 pounds of deveined shrimp (large and peeled)
Pepper
Five tablespoons olive oil
Two tablespoons of lemon juice (fresh)
Half a cucumber (slice into shapes of half-moon)
One avocado (quartered)

Method:

1. In a bowl, place the shrimp and hurl with two tbsps. of oil and half a tsp. each of pepper and salt. Heat a grill pan and on the other hand, brush the pineapple with one tbsp. of oil. Grill the pineapple and shrimp until charred and opaque respectively, in batches on baking sheets (rimmed).
2. Grill the whole thing for about three minutes each side (or for eight minutes if you are using a broiler).
3. In the meantime, use another bowl to whip together the lemon juice, two tbsps. of oil, a quarter tsp. each of pepper and salt and onion. Mix them well.
4. Make even smaller slices of the grilled pineapple, and add onion, cucumber, and shrimp, shake it well to mix. Bend in avocado and watercress.

Meal 2 – 4 pm – Chickpea Pasta Salad

Total Prep & Cooking Time: 10 minutes
Yields: 1 serving
Nutrition Facts: Calories: 377 | Carbs: 50.5g | Protein: 11.3g
| Fat: 8.8g | Fiber: 7g

Ingredients:

Half a cup of baby arugula (chopped)
Two tablespoons each of

- kalamata olives (halved)
- olive oil
- red wine vinegar
- crumbled feta

A quarter cup of canned chickpeas (rinsed)
One cup of cooked pasta (spiral)
A quarter of a small-sized onion (chopped finely)
To taste: salt and pepper
One cup of grape tomatoes (halved)

Method:

1. Add onion, oil, red wine vinegar, and one pinch each of pepper and salt to a quarter portion of the jar. Add the chickpeas and toss them gently to coat well with the ingredients.
2. Crown the mixture with arugula, tomatoes, pasta, feta, and olives. Reverse the jar, allow the contents to settle for two minutes, and let the dressing run over the ingredients properly.

Meal 3 – 6 pm – Rainbow Fruit Parfaits

Total Prep & Cooking Time: 10 minutes
Yields: Four servings
Nutrition Facts: Calories: 146 | Carbs: 26g | Protein: 5g | Fat: 1g
| Fiber: 3g

Ingredients:

Half a cup each of
- Pineapple (chopped)
- Blueberries
- Strawberries (sliced)
- Red grapes (seedless)

Two mandarins (peeled and segmented)
Two kiwis (peeled and chopped)
One cup of vanilla yogurt (Greek)

Method:

1. Summon up the parfaits with layers of oranges, kiwi, grapes, pineapple, strawberries, blueberries, and grapes in four parfait glasses.
2. Crown the glasses with a spoonful of yogurt and enjoy.

Meal 4 – 9 pm – Mango and Roasted Salmon

Total Prep & Cooking Time: 30 minutes
Yields: Four people
Nutrition Facts: Calories: 301 | Carbs: 12g | Protein: 29g
| Fat: 15g | Fiber: 2g

Ingredients:

Four ounces of salmon filets (four pieces)
One jar (seven ounces) of roasted and drained red peppers, sliced
into strips
Two tbsps. of butter (unsalted and divided)
One tbsp. each of

- Water
- Onion (finely chopped)

One tsp. each of

- Jalapeno peppers (minced)
- Cornstarch

Three tbsps. of lime juice (fresh and divided)
One cup of fresh mango, chopped and peeled
To taste: Salt and Pepper

Method:

1. Heat the oven beforehand to cook. Use a section of foil paper to twine around a baking sheet. Spray the cooking utensil with cooking spray (nonstick).
2. You will need a small bowl. Use the small-sized bowl to whip the water and cornstarch together. Combine them well. Set the mixture aside for some time.
3. Turn the oven to medium to high heat and place a skillet on the oven. Take one tbsp. of butter, add it to the skillet and let it melt. Now add onion, and cook for about one minute until you get the fragrance.
4. Add mango, jalapeno, and roasted red peppers and cook. Keep stirring for another two minutes to combine all the ingredients properly. Add the mixture of cornstarch along with two tbsps. of lime juice to the mixture above.
5. Stir the mixture constantly. Cook until the mixture becomes thick. After you know the cooking is done, remove and keep it aside warm.
6. Take a small bowl and add the remaining tbsp. of butter and lime juice to it. Stir it well with the help of a spinner.
7. Put salmon fillets on the baking sheet lined with foil paper. Sprinkle pepper and salt to the filets. Use half of the butter and lime juice (mixture) and brush on one side. Cook this side of the fillet for five minutes. Turn the filet and brush with another half of the mixture. Continue cooking for five to seven minutes. Make sure that the fish is cooked thoroughly and easily flakes.
8. Serve with mango and red pepper sauce and enjoy.

Day 3
Meal 1 – 1 pm – Egg and Cheese Sandwich

Total Prep & Cooking Time: 10 minutes
Yields: 4 Servings
Nutrition Facts: Calories: 326 | Carbs: 30g | Protein: 16g | Fat: 15g | Fiber: 2.3g

Ingredients:

One tablespoon olive oil
Four English muffins (Toasted)
Four eggs (Large)
Two ounces of extra-sharp cheddar cheese (Grated coarsely)
Kosher pepper and salt
Two cups of baby spinach
Four thin slices of ham (optional)

Method:

1. Mix one tablespoon of water and a quarter teaspoon of salt and pepper. Beat the eggs in a bowl with this mixture. Use a large nonstick skillet to heat the oil in medium flame.
2. Add the beaten eggs to the heated oil. Use a rubber spatula to stir the eggs. Stir frequently to get the desired softness. To get eggs of medium softness, cook for two or three minutes.
3. Dollop the eggs at the bottom of the muffin. Use spinach, ham, and cheese as toppings. Repeat the process for each muffin. Make a sandwich with the rest of the muffin top.

Meal 2 – 4 pm – Green Carrot Salad

Total Prep & Cooking Time: 30 minutes
Yields: 4 Servings
Nutrition Facts: Calories: 200 | Carbs: 13g | Protein: 4g | Fat: 15g | Fiber: 4g

Ingredients:

One pound of slim baby carrots – Trimmed and cut into halves vertically, or in quarters, if large
One cup of green goddess dressing
One head Bibb lettuce – Torn and leaves separated
One tablespoon of olive oil

For Green Dressing,
Half cup of mayonnaise
One small clove of garlic
Dash of sugar
A quarter teaspoon of pepper
Half cup of fresh parsley – Loosely packed
Three-quarters teaspoon of salt
A quarter cup of loosely packed fresh basil
Three tablespoons of fresh tarragon
Two tablespoons of sniffed fresh chives
Three-quarters cup of buttermilk
One-third cup of plain Greek Yogurt
Two teaspoons of anchovy paste or four anchovies
One tablespoon of Dijon mustard
Two tablespoons of fresh lemon juice

Method:

1. Heat the oven to four hundred and twenty-five degrees Fahrenheit. In a rimmed baking sheet, add carrots, half a tsp. salt and olive oil. Roast till the edges of the carrot mildly caramelized, turn crispy tender. This takes twenty minutes. Cool the carrots.
2. For Green Goddess dressing, add Greek yogurt, lemon juice, Dijon mustard, a dash of sugar, pepper, salt, buttermilk, mayonnaise, anchovies paste or anchovies and garlic, to a blender. Make a smooth puree. Add chives, parsley, basil, and tarragon. Pulse until the leaves are chopped finely.
3. Place the carrots on the lettuce. Splash the dressing over the carrots. Serve and enjoy.

Meal 3 – 6 pm – Avocado Chips

Total Prep & Cooking Time: 33 minutes
Yields: 24 Chips
Nutrition Facts: Calories: 191 | Carbs: 6g | Protein: 7g | Fat: 16.5g | Fiber: 4g

Ingredients:

A three-quarters cup of parmesan cheese (Grated)
Half a teaspoon of garlic powder
One teaspoon of lemon juice
A large-sized Hass avocado (deseeded and peeled)
A quarter teaspoon of onion powder
One-eighth teaspoon of black pepper

Method:

1. Set the temperature of the oven to three hundred and twenty-five degrees Fahrenheit. Take two half baking sheets. Line them with silicone baking mats. Alternatively, parchment papers can be used.
2. Puree the avocado by mashing it with a spoon in a medium-sized bowl. When completely pureed, add garlic powder, black pepper, lemon juice, cheese, and onion powder. Mix everything to blend thoroughly.
3. On the prepared baking sheet place a heaping teaspoon of this batter. Repeat with the rest, and each dollop should have a gap of three inches. In the half sheet pan of eighteen by thirteen inches, a dozen chips would fit.
4. Cut the parchment paper to make it fit into a pan. Place this on the dollops.
5. Take off this paper gently, and any batter stuck to it should be placed back on the rounds.
6. Bake the rounds till the cheese turns brown or for fifteen minutes. Use a thin cookie spatula and gently turn the chips to the other side. Cook for another two minutes.
7. Cool the chips because it helps in making the chips crispy.

Meal 4 – 9 pm – Rosemary Chicken Thighs

Total Prep & Cooking Time: 1 Hour 15 minutes
Yields: 4 Servings

Ingredients:

A cup of quinoa
A quarter tsp. of cayenne pepper
Two lemons – zested, cut into halves
Four chicken thighs – with bones and skin, and trimmed off the extra
fat if required
Kosher salt
One garlic clove (Minced)
Freshly ground black pepper – to taste
One small head broccoli (Cut into florets)
A handful of fresh parsley
Two sprigs of fresh Rosemary (leaves taken off from the stem)
Two tbsp. of extra virgin olive oil (Divided)
Half a cup of frozen peas
One and Three-quarters cup of chicken broth

Method:

1. Blend parsley, rosemary, lemon zest, cayenne pepper, salt, and pepper in a mini food processor till the herbs are chopped finely. Spread the herb mixture on both sides of the chicken thighs. Refrigerate for thirty minutes. You can refrigerate up to twelve hours.
2. Heat the oven to four hundred and fifty degrees Fahrenheit.
3. Heat one tbsp. olive oil on high heat in a pan. Roast the chicken with the skin down till it turns golden, and this takes five minutes. Flip and cook for two minutes. Take off the chicken and remove excess fat.
4. To the pan, add half a cup of chicken broth, chicken thighs, broccoli florets, and chicken thighs.
5. Bake the chicken up to twenty minutes in the preheated oven. Cover the chicken pieces with foil on a plate. Keep aside lemon and broccoli.
6. Cover the pan after adding the remaining chicken broth, garlic, and quinoa. Bake again for twenty minutes.
7. When the liquid is absorbed fully, take off the pan and add chicken thighs, broccoli, frozen peas, and chicken thighs. Bake again for five minutes. Remove and use a fork to fluff the quinoa. Add a few drops of roasted lemon juice just before serving.

Day 4
Meal 1 – 1 pm – Healthy Burrito

Total prep and cooking time: Thirty minutes
Yields: 1 serving
Nutritional facts: Calorie: 321 | Protein: 20.3g | Fat: 11.4g |Carbs: 36.9g | Fiber: 3.7g

Ingredients:

Four eggs (large)
Half a cup each of

- Yellow onion, diced
- Red bell pepper, diced

Four large tortillas
Eight egg whites
Half a teaspoon of onion powder
Four ounces of diced red potatoes
Two cups of chopped spinach
One teaspoon of garlic powder
Four Sugarhouse Maple Breakfast chicken sausages
Salt and pepper

For toppings,
Salsa
Avocado or Guacamole slices
Shredded cheese
Fresh cilantro

Method:

1. Sauté the potatoes in a large skillet for about three-five minutes until they get softened and then add in the chopped chicken sausages, onion, and bell pepper. After cooking those for a couple of minutes, add in the spinach. When the veggies get soft and sausages turn brown, add the egg whites, eggs and seasoning.
2. Fill the tortillas with about one-fourth of the mixture. Fold in the sides over the filling and tuck in the edges as you roll it.
3. Add the burritos in another hot skillet with the seam side down. Cook them covered for three minutes until the bottom turns golden. Flip them over and cook them covered for a few more minutes until they turn golden.

Meal 2 – 4 pm – Green and Herb Salad

Total Prep & Cooking Time: 10 minutes
Yields: 6 servings
Nutrition facts: Calories: 125 | Protein: 3g | Fat: 10g | Carbs: 6g
| Fiber: 2g

Ingredients:

One cup of shelled edamame
Six cups of mixed spring greens, torn
One-fourth cup of olive oil
Two cups of mixed herbs, chopped
One tablespoon of lemon juice
One teaspoon of honey
Two tablespoons of Dijon mustard
One shallot (small), finely chopped
Salt and pepper

For serving,
Edible flowers
Soft-cooked eggs

Method:

1. Take a large bowl and add the mixed greens and herbs.
2. Fold in the edamame.
3. Mix the olive oil, Dijon mustard, honey, and lemon juice together in a bowl and season with one-fourth teaspoon of salt and pepper. Add the chopped shallots and stir.
4. Toss the salad gently with the dressing.
5. You can add the eggs and edible flowers as a topping.

Meal 3 – 6 pm – Roasted Garlic Hummus

Total Prep & Cooking Time: 1 Hour
Yields: 1 1/3 Cups
Nutrition Facts: Calories: 95 | Carbs: 6g | Protein: 1g | Fat: 8g
| Fiber: 2g

Ingredients:

Four tbsps. of extra virgin olive oil (Divided)
Three tbsp. and one and a half tsp. of fresh lemon juice (from a large juicy lemon)
A can of chickpeas of fifteen and a half oz. (Rinsed and Drained)
Two heads of garlic
Two tbsp. of Tahini
A three-quarter tsp. of salt
Sumac powder, parsley (chopped), and additional extra virgin olive oil – for garnishing and optional

Method:

1. Set the temperature of the oven to three hundred and fifty degrees Fahrenheit. From the whole heads of garlic, remove the papery skin that is extra by rubbing. Using a serrated knife cut the tips of each clove of garlic. Take a small baking dish and lay the garlic with the root side down. You can use a sheet of aluminum foil. On the cut end of the garlic, dash two tbsps. of oil. Crimp the foil to close the garlic, or if using a baking dish, cover it with a foil. Now roast the garlic till the cloves become soft and release the aroma. Unpack the foil and let the garlic cloves cool.

2. Remove the papery skin by squeezing the garlic cloves. Throw off the skin, and in a food processor, add the cloves. Chickpeas, two tbsps. of oil, tahini, salt, and lemon juice should be added to the food processor. Puree till the contents become smooth. Garnish with parsley, sumac powder, and olive oil, if preferred.

Meal 4 – 9 pm – Orange Chicken Stir Fry

Total Prep & Cooking Time: 1 hour
Yields: 4 servings
Nutrition facts: Calories: 391 | Protein: 30.3g | Fat: 17.8g
| Carbs: 33.4g | Fiber: 4g

Ingredients:

For the cauliflower rice,
One head of cauliflower
Salt
Pepper
One tablespoon coconut oil

For the sauce,
One tablespoon arrowroot or cornstarch
Two tablespoons of honey
Half tablespoon of ginger, freshly grated
Zest from one large orange
Three tablespoons of soy sauce
Half teaspoon of chili flakes
Three-fourth of a cup of orange juice

For the stir-fry,
One pound of chicken breast (skinless and boneless), diced into bite-sized pieces
Half white onion, diced into chunks
Eight ounces of fresh green beans, cut into two-inch pieces
1 ½ tablespoon sesame oil
Three cloves of garlic, minced
Half cup of cashews
One red bell pepper (large), sliced
Salt and pepper

To garnish,
Sesame seeds (toasted)
Green onion

Method:

1. For the cauliflower rice, pulse the florets in a food processor until it becomes rice-like. Squeeze out the moisture using a clean dish towel and set aside.
2. For the sauce, whisk all the ingredients in a bowl until the cornstarch dissolves.
3. Add a teaspoon of toasted sesame oil in a heated skillet and add in the chicken and salt and pepper. Cook for five to six minutes until the chicken is fully cooked and no longer pink. Transfer the cooked chicken into a bowl and keep it aside.
4. Add half teaspoon of sesame oil in the hot skillet. Sauté the onions for about two minutes until they turn translucent. Then add the garlic, green beans, bell pepper, and cashews and cook for four-six minutes.
5. In another skillet, add half teaspoon of coconut oil and cauliflower rice and cook for five minutes. Stir occasionally and season with salt and pepper.
6. Add the orange sauce into the pan, stirring frequently. Stir in the chicken. Allow the sauce to simmer for about three minutes so that it gets thicker.
7. Add the green onions and toasted sesame seeds as a topping and serve with the cauliflower rice.

Day 5
Meal 1 – 1 pm – Watermelon Cucumber Smoothie

Total Prep & Cooking Time: 5 minutes
Yields: 4 servings
Nutrition facts: Calories: 63 | Protein: 1.5g | Fat: 0.5g | Carbs: 16g | Fiber: 2g

Ingredients:

Three Persian cucumbers (medium-sized), washed and chopped
One cup of ice
Half cup of fresh mint leaves
One-third cup of lime juice (freshly squeezed)
Five cups of watermelon (seedless), diced into chunks
Pomegranate seeds for garnishing (optional)

Method:

1. Blend the watermelon, cucumber, mint leaves, lime juice, and ice in a blender until you get a smooth mixture.
2. Pour the smoothie into four separate glasses. Garnish them with pomegranate seeds and mint leaves and serve immediately.

Meal 2 – 4 pm – Chicken and Red Plum Salad

Total Prep & Cooking Time: 20 minutes
Yields: 4 servings
Nutritional facts: Calories: 355 | Protein: 38g | Fat: 16.5g
| Carbs: 12g | Fiber: 3g

Ingredients:

Four red plums, sliced into one-inch wedges
Six cups of baby arugula
Half cup of roughly chopped fresh dill
Two scallions, thinly sliced
Two tablespoons + one teaspoon of olive oil
46 ounces of chicken breasts (boneless, skinless)
One-fourth cup of chopped roasted almonds
One-fourth teaspoon each of salt and pepper

Method:

1. Heat the grill to medium.
2. Rub a teaspoon of olive oil on the chicken breast and season with salt and pepper. Add the red plums in a large bowl and toss them with a tablespoon of oil and salt and pepper.
3. Grill the chicken for five-seven minutes on each side until it gets cooked. Transfer the cooked chicken onto a cutting board. Allow it to rest for five minutes before slicing into pieces.
4. Grill the plums for two-three minutes per side until they get just charred. Transfer into a bowl and toss with the scallions and oil.
5. Add the chicken along with its juices into the bowl and toss to mix everything together. Fold in the arugula, chopped almonds, and dill.

Meal 3 – 6 pm – Berry Parfait

Total Prep & Cooking Time: 15 minutes
Yields: Four servings
Nutritional facts: Calories: 384 | Protein: 18g | Fat: 9g | Carbs: 59g
| Fiber: 7g

Ingredients:

Three cups of plain yogurt (2%)
Two cups of blueberries, raspberries and/or strawberries
One cup of rolled oats (large flake)
Three tablespoons of brown sugar (granulated/packed)
One tablespoon of flax seeds (optional)
One teaspoon of vanilla extract
One-fourth cup of almonds/pecans/walnuts, chopped

Method:

1. Heat a skillet over medium heat. Add the oats and nuts into the skillet and toast them for two to three minutes, stirring constantly until it turns golden and fragrant.
2. Transfer the toasted oats immediately into a bowl and allow it to cool. Add the flax seeds (optional).
3. Whisk the yogurt, sugar, and vanilla extract together in a bowl.
4. Add the toasted oats mixture, yogurt, and berries in alternate layers in four separate reusable containers with lids. Refrigerate the closed containers for at least eight hours or up to two days.

Meal 4 – 9 pm – Swedish Meatballs

Total Prep & Cooking Time: 45 minutes
Yields: 4 servings
Nutritional facts: Calories: 459 | Protein: 45g | Fat: 22g
| Carbs: 23g | Fiber: 5g

Ingredients:

For the meatballs,
One egg
One pound lean turkey (ground)
One-fourth cup each of
- Panko
- Almond milk (unsweetened)

One teaspoon of dill (dried)
One tablespoon of parsley (dried)
Half teaspoon of kosher salt
1 ½ teaspoon of onion flakes (dried)
One-fourth teaspoon each of
- Black pepper
- Ground allspice

For the white sauce,
One cup each of
- Low-sodium chicken broth
- Almond milk (unsweetened)

Half cup of plain Greek yogurt (non-fat)
One-third cup of shallot/onion, minced
Two tablespoons of freshly chopped flat-leaf parsley
One teaspoon each of
- Worcestershire
- Fresh thyme, chopped

Pepper
Kosher salt

Method:

For meatballs,

1. Whisk the egg, panko, almond milk, and spices together in a bowl.
2. Add the ground turkey into it and combine using your hands.
3. Make approximately 20 meatballs using a 1 ½ tablespoon cookie scoop. You can also eyeball the amount.
4. Cook the meatballs in a heated skillet for about eight minutes until they get brown on all sides and properly cooked.
5. Transfer the cooked meatballs into a plate and keep them covered with a foil to keep them warm.

For the white sauce,

1. Heat some olive oil over medium heat in the same skillet.
2. Add the minced onions and sauté for two minutes until they get softened.
3. Add the flour and whisk until it gets smooth and then cook for a minute.
4. Pour the almond milk and chicken broth slowly, whisking continuously.
5. Season with salt and pepper and add the fresh thyme and Worcestershire.
6. Simmer the mixture while whisking it continuously until it thickens.
7. When the sauce thickens, remove from heat and add the Greek yogurt slowly and whisk until smooth.
8. Add half of the chopped parsley.
9. Transfer the meatballs into the sauce and garnish with the remaining chopped parsley.

Day 6
Meal 1 – 1 pm – Ultimate Green Smoothie

Total Prep & Cooking Time: 5 minutes
Yields: One
Nutrition facts: Calories: 238 | Protein: 4g | Fat: 12g | Carbs: 13g | Fiber: 9g

Ingredients:

One apple (chopped)
A two-third cup of apple juice
A quarter avocado (sliced)
Four florets of broccoli (frozen)

Method:

Mix all the ingredients so that they combine together and enjoy.

Meal 2 – 4 pm – Lentil Wraps

Total Prep & Cooking Time: 50 minutes
Yields: Four servings
Nutrition Facts: Calories:381 | Carbs: 43.5g | Protein:18.4g
| Fat: 13.9g | Fiber: 12.1g

Ingredients:

One tsp. each of
- olive oil
- cumin
- coriander

One cup of lentils (dried)
To taste: Salt
Pepper (cracked)
One to two cloves of garlic (minced finely)
One tbsp. olive oil
Two tbsps. each of
- tahini paste
- lemon juice (fresh)

Half a tsp. of kosher salt
Three tbsps. of water (warm)
One tsp. of Sriracha sauce
Three cups of scallions and cilantro (chopped)
Warm tortillas (4 *12 inches)
Two tbsps. of sunflower, toasted (optional)
One and a half cups each of
- cabbage (shredded)
- carrots (shredded)

Half avocado, sliced (optional)

Method:

1. Light your oven. Place a pot with some water poured in it. Cook the lentils firmly. After some time, drain the excess water from lentils and flavor with olive oil, cumin, salt, and coriander.
2. While the lentils are being cooked, you can use the time to make the tahini sauce. For that, you will need a small bowl and a fork to whisk the ingredients. Mix warm water, lemon juice, salt, tahini paste, olive oil, garlic, pepper, and Sriracha sauce. Combine until the mixture is creamy.
3. Prepare all the vegetables.
4. Heat the tortillas over a gas stove on medium flame to make the wraps. Flip and turn the tortillas until they are smooth and warm (or use a toaster to toast the tortillas). If you are using a toaster, make sure to not over toast to prevent it from becoming tough.
5. Roll up cilantro, veggies, scallions, and dived lentils like a burrito.
6. Cut the roll-ups in half (at diagonal).
7. Serve with spicy tahini sauce.

Meal 3 – 6 pm – Keto Berry Mousse

Total Prep & Cooking Time: 10 minutes
Yields: Eight servings
Nutrition Facts: Calories: 225 | Carbs: 3g | Protein: 2g | Fat: 26g
| Fiber: 1g

Ingredients:

Half lemon (zested)
Three ounces of raspberries or strawberries or blueberries (fresh)
A quarter teaspoon of vanilla extract
Two ounces of pecans (chopped)
Two cups of whipping cream (heavy)

Method:

1. For preparing the mousse you need to have a small-sized bowl and hand mixer.
2. Use the bowl to place the cream in it and whisk the cream with the help of a hand mixer until the cream forms soft summits.
3. After you are done with whipping the cream, add vanilla and lemon zest to the bowl.
4. Now you need to add the berries (strawberry or blueberry or raspberry) to the cream (whipped) and stir the mixture thoroughly.
5. Wrap up the mouth of the bowl with the help of plastic and put it inside the refrigerator. Let the mixture sit for about three hours to prepare a smooth mousse.
6. Enjoy the mousse immediately for a less smooth consistency.

Meal 4 – 9 pm – Sweet and Spicy Chicken

Total Prep & Cooking Time: 1 hour
Yields: Four people
Nutrition Facts: Calories: 560 | Carbs: 27g | Protein: 57g | Fat: 22g | Fiber: 1g

Ingredients:

One pound of asparagus (halved and trimmed)
One pound of sweet potatoes (cut into chunks of one inch size)
Half a teaspoon of ginger (freshly grated)
One tablespoon each of

- olive oil
- coriander seeds (crushed)

Cilantro, fresh (for the purpose of garnishing)
Two teaspoons of pure honey
A quarter cup of chili-garlic sauce
One whole chicken (four lb.) spatchcocked
One teaspoon of lime zest and two tbsps. of lime juice
Kosher salt and pepper (freshly ground)

Method:

1. Set temperature of the oven to 425 degrees Fahrenheit and preheat. You will require a baking sheet (rimmed). Place the chicken on the rimmed baking sheet (breast on the upper side). Season the chicken breast with pepper and salt.
2. Use a small mixing bowl to combine lime zest, chili-garlic sauce, lime juice, and garlic. Transfer half of the mixture to another bowl (about three tbsps.) and pour some honey in it. Stir it well. Set the mixture aside for some time. Brush mixture on both sides of chicken and let it roast for about twenty minutes.
3. Use another bowl to toss the potatoes, coriander, and oil together with a spoon. Season the mixture with pepper and salt. Scatter the mixture around chicken. Roast the chicken for about eighteen to twenty minutes. A thermometer (instant-read), when placed inside the thickest portion of the thigh, should register 168 degrees Fahrenheit.
4. Roast for ten minutes until the asparagus is soft. Allow chicken to stay for five minutes prior to carving.
5. Serve the chicken with vegetables along the side. Enjoy with garnished cilantro and remaining sauce.

Day 7
Meal 1 – 1 pm – Instant Pot Frittata

Total Prep & Cooking Time: 30 minutes
Yields: Four servings
Nutrition Facts: Calories: 195 | Carbs: 5g | Protein: 14g | Fat: 12g | Fiber: 1g

Ingredients:

Three green onions (chopped)
Black pepper
Six eggs
Two oz. of cheddar cheese (shredded, half a cup)
Eight oz. of broccoli florets (chopped finely)
Half a tsp. of sea salt (fine)

Method:

1. Take a large-sized bowl and beat the eggs into the bowl along with several crushes of black pepper and salt. Add green onion, cheddar cheese and broccoli (chopped) to the bowl and mix thoroughly to combine them well.
2. You will require a seven-inch pan. Grease the inner surface of the pan with a handsome amount of oil. Let the egg mixture to flow in the pan.
3. Take an instant pot and discharge one cup of water in it. Fit a trivet over the instant pot, so the pan lies above the water.
4. Pour the frittata mixture in the pan and place it on top of trivet, cover the pan with a lid. The valve for releasing the steam should be moved to sealing. Cook the frittata at high pressure for about ten minutes.
5. After the broiling cycle is over, let it release the pressure naturally for about ten minutes (specifically speaking, the set up for ten minutes without doing anything to it). Once the screen of your machine reads L0:10, it is time to start the process of venting. This will release the excess pressure.
6. You can safely remove the lid after floating valve drops.

7. Transfer the frittata pan using oven mitts. There is nothing to get shocked by noticing water droplets on baked eggs. They will evaporate as soon as it cools.
8. Make four slices of the frittata and enjoy it warm.
9. Store the leftovers in an airtight container in a fridge for up to five days.

Meal 2 – 4 pm – Shaved Brussels Sprouts Salad

Total Prep & Cooking Time: 15 minutes
Yields: Eight servings
Nutrition Facts: Calories: 215 | Carbs: 18g | Protein: 5g | Fat: 14g | Fiber: 3g

Ingredients:

For dressing,
One clove of garlic (minced)
One tbsp. each of
- Lemon juice (fresh)
- Maple syrup (pure)

One-third cup of olive oil
Two tbsps. apple cider, vinegar
Two tsps. of Dijon mustard
To taste: Kosher salt and black pepper

For salad,
One-third cup of parmesan cheese (shredded or shaved)
One pound of Brussels sprouts (ends trimmed)
Half a cup each of
- Sunflower seeds
- Cranberries (dried)

Black pepper
One honey-crisp apple, large (chopped)

Method:

1. We will be making the maple mustard dressing at first. Take a mixing bowl (large) to whip together the lemon juice, pure maple syrup, olive oil, apple cider vinegar, garlic, and mustard. Season the mixture with ground pepper and kosher salt. Set the mixture aside.
2. Then you need to cut off the sprouts. With the help of a food processor (which has slicing attachment), pulse the sprouts until they become thin slices. (A sharp knife or a mandolin can also be used).
3. Put the Brussels sprouts (shredded) in a bowl and add dried cranberries, parmesan cheese, chopped apple and sunflower seeds to it.
4. Drizzle salad with dressing and toss the mixture well.
5. Serve with seasoned salt and pepper.

Meal 3 – 6 pm – Coconut Mocha Frappe

Total Preparation time: 5 minutes
Yields: One
Nutrition Facts: Calories: 120 | Carbs: 2g | Protein: 0g | Fat: 10g | Fiber: 0g

Ingredients:

One drop of coconut extract
One packet of instant coffee (about two teaspoons)
One packet of stevia (three and a half ounces)
Half a teaspoon of cocoa powder (unsweetened)
Two cups of coconut milk (unsweetened)

Method:

1. Add all raw ingredients in a large cup.
2. Stir all the ingredients well (there is nothing to worry about if they do not assemble together properly).
3. Use a shallow bowl (freezer safe) to place the mixture. Use a fork to scrape down the mixture in the bowl after every two hours.
4. Once the mixture is frozen, leave it on the counter until you take a softened pinch out of the bowl.
5. Put the mixture in the blender and let it process.

Meal 4 – 9 pm – Sheet Pan Shrimp Fajitas

Total Prep & Cooking Time: 30 minutes
Yields: Eight servings
Nutrition facts: Calories: 100| Carbs: 4.9g | Protein: 14.2g
| Fat: 2.5g | Fiber: 0.6g

Ingredients:

One bell pepper, red in color (cut into strips)
One tbsp. of olive oil
One jalapeno pepper (cut into rings)
One bell pepper yellow in color, (cut into strips)
One and a half lb. of shrimp, raw (deveined and peeled)
One oz. of fajita for seasoning
One red onion (make strips)

Method:

1. Set temperature of the oven to 230 degrees Celsius and preheat.
2. Use a large bowl to mix fajita (seasoning) and olive oil. Add shrimp to the bowl and mix all of them well so that the ingredients coat the shrimp properly.
3. Use a baking sheet to spread out shrimp (seasoned), red bell pepper, onion (red), yellow bell pepper, and jalapeno pepper evenly on the baking sheet.
4. Roast shrimp for ten minutes until opaque.
5. Cook the pepper mixture for three minutes and enjoy the roasted shrimp.

Day 8
Meal 1 – 1 pm – Ham and Egg Muffins

Total Prep & Cooking Time: 35 minutes
Yields: Six servings
Nutrition Facts: Calories: 260 | Carbs: 4.9g | Protein: 27.9g
| Fat: 14.2g | Fiber; 0g

Ingredients:

Half a teaspoon of kosher salt
Half a cup of cheddar cheese, white and shredded (or mozzarella cheese)
A quarter cup of onion (diced)
Twelve slices of deli ham, thin
Cooking spray, nonstick
Ten eggs (large)
One medium-sized tomato (chopped)
Three fourth cup of fresh spinach (lightly packed and chopped)
To taste – Black pepper (freshly ground)

Method:

1. Set the temperature of the oven to 350 degrees Fahrenheit because the first step is preheating.
2. Since we are making twelve muffins, take a pan that can accommodate them. Coat the muffin pan using cooking spray (non-stick one).
3. Use the ham slices to line the muffin cups. Divide the onions, cheese, tomatoes, and spinach among the cups, evenly.
4. Utilize a large-sized bowl to beat the eggs and whisk them with the desired amount of salt. Sprinkle black pepper as you require to. Blend them properly.
5. Now, pour egg (mixture) to muffin cups evenly. The egg mixture can be easily scooped from the bowl with a ladle.
6. Once ready, bake the ingredients in muffin cups for twenty minutes. Make sure the tops are cooked well after twenty minutes. If not, place the muffin pan under the broiler for another minute.
7. Let the muffins cool for about five minutes and remove by circling a knife around muffins to detach from the cups and serve them hot.

Meal 2 – 4 pm – Classic Cobb Salad

Total Prep & Cooking Time: 35 minutes
Yields: Four servings
Nutrition Facts: Calories: 913 | Carbs: 31g | Protein: 53g | Fat: 66g | Fiber: 0g

Ingredients:

One clove of garlic (crushed)
Half a tsp. each of
- Black pepper (freshly ground)
- Dijon mustard

A quarter tsp. of salt
One tsp. of Worcestershire sauce
Four oz. of Roquefort cheese, crumbled
A quarter cup of red wine vinegar
Two medium-sized tomatoes, chopped (ripe)
Four cups of chicken (cooked and diced)
Three hard-boiled eggs, peeled and chopped
Two avocados, pitted, diced and peeled (ripe)
One romaine lettuce (head)
Eight slices of bacon

Method:

1. Fry bacon pieces until they are crispy. Use paper towels for draining the excess oil. Allow them to cool down so that they can be handled and crumbled. Set them aside.
2. Form a layer of lettuce leaves on serving plates. Line the bacon, avocado, Roquefort cheese, eggs, chicken, and tomatoes (in straight rows) on top of the bed of lettuce. Cover the plates completely.
3. Take a bowl and whip the vinegar, garlic, pepper, mustard, Worcestershire sauce, and salt together. Mix them well. Slowly dribble olive oil over the mixture, whisking continuously, to prepare the dressing.
4. Dribble the dressing slowly over salad. Serve and enjoy without delay.

Meal 3 – 6 pm – Mixed Berries

Total Prep & Cooking Time: 5 minutes
Yields: 1 serving
Nutrition Facts: Calories: 70 | Carbs: 17g | Protein: 1g | Fat: 0.5g
| Fiber: 5g

Ingredients:

Eight oz. each of
- Fresh blueberries
- Fresh blackberries

Two pints of fresh strawberries
Two tbsps. of lime juice
Four oz. of fresh raspberries
Half a cup of pomegranate seeds
One tbsp. of honey

Method:

Mix everything together in a bowl and toss well.

Meal 4 – 9 pm – Low Carb Beef Chili

Total Prep & Cooking Time: 1 hour 10 minutes
Yields: Six servings
Nutrition Facts: Calories: 357 | Crabs: 920mg | Protein: 33g
|Fat: 21g | Fiber: 9g

Ingredients:

Two tbsps. of chili powder
Fifteen oz. of canned tomatoes (diced)
One clove of garlic (minced)
One green pepper (diced)
One and a half lbs. beef (ground)
One tsp. each of

- Cumin
- Salt

Two cups of beef broth
A quarter cup of tomato paste
One jalapeno (minced)
One yellow onion (diced)

Method:

1. Add ground beef, bell pepper, and onion to a deep pot. Put the oven to medium heat and cook. After the meat is cooked, drain the fat.
2. Add garlic, tomatoes, chili powder, jalapeno, tomato paste, beef broth, salt, and cumin. Stir to mix. Let it boil. Simmer for twenty minutes for better taste.
3. Serve with cheddar cheese (shredded) and cream and enjoy.

Day 9
Meal 1 – 1 pm – Baked Avocado Boats

Total Prep & Cooking Time: 40 minutes
Yields: 4 Servings
Nutrition Facts: Calories: 220 | Carbs: 6g | Protein: 10g | Fat: 18g | Fiber: 5g

Ingredients:

Four large eggs
Three slices of bacon
Black pepper – freshly ground
Kosher salt
Two ripe avocados – pitted and cut into halves
Chives – Freshly chopped to garnish

Method:

1. Heat the oven. Set three hundred and fifty Fahrenheit. Scoop out from each half of the avocado, flesh of about one tbsp.
2. Keep the scooped avocado in a baking dish, and break the eggs one by one into it. Place one yolk per avocado. Try to scoop the egg whites as much as possible into the avocado halves. Ensure there is no spilling.
3. For seasoning, add pepper and salt. Bake the avocados for twenty to twenty-five minutes. The whites should be set, and the yolk should not be runny. If avocados turn brown, use a foil to cover them.
4. Cook bacon in a large skillet in medium flame. Cook for eight minutes till the bacon is crispy. Line a plate with a paper towel, and place the bacon on it to chop.
5. Serve avocados with the bacon and chives topping.

Meal 2 – 4 pm – Cinnamon Almond Butter Smoothie

Total Prep & Cooking Time: 2 minutes
Yields: 1 Serving
Nutrition Facts: Calories: 326 | Carbs: 11g | Protein: 19g
| Fat: 27g | Fiber: 5g

Ingredients:

One scoop of collagen peptides
Half a teaspoon of cinnamon
Fifteen drops of liquid stevia
One-eighth teaspoon of almond extract
One-eighth teaspoon of salt
Two tablespoons of almond butter
One and a half cup of unsweetened nut milk
Two tablespoons of golden flax meal
Six to eight ice cubes

Method:

1. Mix collagen peptides, cinnamon, liquid stevia, unsweetened milk, almond butter, golden flax meal, salt, almond extract, and ice cubes in a blender.
2. Blend for thirty seconds to get a smooth consistency. Serve.

Meal 3 – 6 pm – Melon, Cucumber, and Feta Skewers

Total Prep & Cooking Time: 10 minutes
Yields: 20 Servings
Nutrition Facts: Calories: 40 | Carbs: 3g | Protein: 3g | Fat: 1.5g
| Fiber: 0g

Ingredients:

Twenty seedless watermelon cubes of one inch each (Or about two and a half cups)
Twenty cubes of seedless cucumber of one inch each
Twenty cubes of feta cheese of one inch each (or about eight ounces)
Cracked black pepper – to taste
Pink Himalayan salt – to taste

Method:

1. Thread the following into the wooden skewer – one melon cube, one feta cheese cube, and one cucumber cube. Repeat the same for all the twenty pieces.
2. Dash pepper and salt on these.

Meal 4 – 9 pm – Greek Salmon Salad

Total Prep & Cooking Time: 25 minutes
Yields: 4 Servings
Nutrition Facts: Calories: 780 | Carbs: 17g | Protein: 86g
| Fat: 49.9g | Fiber: 4.3g

Ingredients:

One clove of garlic (Minced)
Three tbsp. of red wine vinegar
Three-quarters tsp. of dried oregano
A quarter tsp. of freshly ground black pepper
A quarter cup of cold water
Two medium heads of butter lettuce (Boston or Bibb) of one lb. - torn into pieces of bite-sized
Four salmon fillets (of 6 oz.), removed off the skin
Two medium tomatoes, each cut into pieces of one inch
Half cup of pitted kalamata olives, cut into halves vertically
Two tablespoons of lemon juice – freshly squeezed (from one lemon)
Half a tsp. of kosher salt
Half small-sized red onion, sliced into thin pieces
One medium English cucumber- quartered vertically, and cut into half-inch pieces
Four oz. of feta cheese (about one cup, Crumbled)
A quarter cup of olive oil

Method:

1. Preheat the oven to four hundred and twenty-five Fahrenheit. Keep the rack in the middle. Meanwhile, marinate the salmon and soak the red onions.

2. In a large bowl, combine vinegar, garlic, oregano, salt, olive oil, lemon juice, and pepper. Whisk thoroughly. In a baking dish, add three tbsp. of the vinaigrette. Choose a baking dish large enough to hold all the pieces of salmon together in a single layer. Place the salmons in the baking dish. Coat the salmon with the vinaigrette, by turning it gently a few times. Make an even coat. Place the baking dish in the refrigerator, after covering it. In a small bowl, add water and soak the onions to make them less potent. Leave aside for ten minutes. After ten minutes, drain the water and discard it.

3. Remove the salmon from the refrigerator, and roast in the oven. They should be cooked enough to flake easily. This can take about eight to twelve minutes. In the mid of the thickest fillet, the instant-read thermometer should read a hundred and twenty to hundred and thirty Fahrenheit. If you need a well-done salmon, then go for a temperature of hundred and thirty-five to hundred and forty-five degrees Fahrenheit. Cooking time varies based on the thickness of the fillets. Make up the salad while the fillets are cooked.

4. In the vinaigrette bowl, add olives, red onion, cucumber, tomato, and lettuce. Mix to get an even coat. Take four plates or shallow bowls. Place the cooked salmon fillet on each salad. Dash feta on top and serve immediately.

Day 10
Meal 1 – 1 pm – Cauliflower Crusted Quiche

Total Prep & Cooking Time: 1 hour 20 minutes
Yields: 8 quiches
Nutrition Facts: Calories: 219 | Carbs: 11g | Protein: 16g | Fat: 12g | Fiber: 4g

Ingredients:

Four cups of baby spinach (one hundred and sixty gram)
Half a tbsp. of olive oil
Half a cup of feta cheese, crumbled (fifty gram)
Six eggs (divided)
A quarter tsp. of garlic powder
One cauliflower (cut into florets)
Four green onions (chopped)
Eight asparagus, spears (cut into pieces of one inch each)
Half a tsp. of pepper
Half a cup each of
- Milk
- Parmesan cheese, grated (fifty-five grams)

Three-fourth tsp. of salt (divided)

Method:

1. Set temp of oven to 220 degrees Celsius and preheat.
2. Add cauliflower to the bowl of the food processor and let it pulse until they crumble. Microwave the cauliflower for about five minutes and let it cool. Squeeze out excess liquid from cauliflower using a towel.
3. Add one egg, garlic powder, cauliflower, parmesan cheese, and a quarter tsp. of salt to a bowl.
4. Use a tart plate and press the crust mixture on it.
5. Bake for about eighteen minutes until it becomes golden. Set it aside. Let it cool.
6. Reduce the temp of the oven to 190 degrees Celsius.
7. Whisk the remaining eggs, feta cheese (crumbled), pepper, milk, and half tsp of salt in another bowl. Mix them properly.
8. In a medium skillet pour olive oil and heat on medium flame. Add the pieces of asparagus and cook until it turns slightly tender. Add spinach to it and cook until it wilts.
9. Place spinach and asparagus mixture on the base of cauliflower crust and place egg and cheese mixture over it. Sprinkle with onions (green).
10. Bake for about forty-five minutes. Let it cool for another fifteen minutes.
11. Serve and enjoy.

Meal 2 – 4 pm – Instant Pot Chicken Soup

Total Prep & Cooking Time: 1 hour 5 minutes
Yields: Eight bowls of soup
Nutrition Facts: Calories: 182 | Carbs: 7.2g | Protein: 20g | Fat: 8g
| Fiber: 2g

Ingredients:

Half a teaspoon each of
- Rosemary (dried)
- Black pepper (ground)
- Sea salt

Three cloves of garlic (minced)
One and a half cups of cauliflower (chopped)
Two medium-sized carrots (chopped)
A small onion (diced)
One and a quarter pounds of boneless chicken thighs (skinless)
Nine cups chicken broth (or bone stock)
One teaspoon of thyme (dried)
One cup of green beans (sliced into pieces of one inch)
Four stalks of celery (chopped)
One red pepper (diced)
One tablespoon of avocado (or olive oil)

Method:

1. Heat instant pot (o sauté mode). Add some oil to it. Season the chicken thighs with pepper and salt. Once hot, let the chicken thighs (both the sides) to sear until browned. Remove from pot and set it aside.
2. Deglaze the instant pot with a half cup of chicken broth while the machine is still on.
3. Use a spoon (wooden) to scrape off the little pieces of chicken stuck to the side of the pot. Place chicken thighs inside the pot again after shutting it off.
4. Add vegetables (chopped) along with thyme, chicken broth, rosemary, and garlic to the pot. (Be careful to not pour chicken broth more than max fill line).
5. Cover with the lid of the pot and turn the valve (steam release) to seal.
6. Let the chicken cook for twenty-five minutes on high pressure, and once the cooking is done, quick release following the precautions.
7. Shred the chicken using forks, stir into soup and serve warm.

Meal 3 – 6 pm – Raw Kale Salad

Total Prep & Cooking Time: 20 minutes
Yields: Two to Four bowls
Nutrition Facts: Calories: 126 | Carbs: 3g | Protein: 3g | Fat: 12g
| Fiber: 0g

Ingredients:

One-eighth tsp. of sea salt
Two tbsps. each of
- Lemon juice
- Walnut oil
- Olive oil

One shallot (chopped finely)
A quarter cup of hard cheese (finely grated)
One bunch of kale (sliced very thinly)

Method:

1. Chop the kale into small pieces. Place the kale pieces in a salad bowl (large-sized).
2. In another small-sized bowl, mix the salt, lemon juice, and shallot. Combine them properly. Let the mixture settle for about ten minutes for a mellow flavor of the shallot.
3. Add the cheese (grated) and whisk in oil.
4. Pour the dressing on top of the kale pieces and toss the mixture well. Add the excess cheese over the salad and serve.

Meal 4 – 9 pm – Almond Crusted Cod

Total Prep & Cooking Time: 22 minutes
Yields: Four cods' filets
Nutrition Facts: Calories: 219 | Carbs: 4g | Protein: 23g | Fat: 13g
| Fiber: 1g

Ingredients:

Four teaspoons of Dijon mustard
One tablespoon each of
- Olive oil
- Dill

Four cod filets
One teaspoon chili spice
Half a cup of almonds, crushed
To taste: pepper and salt
One medium lemon

Method:

1. Set the temperature of the oven to 400 degrees Fahrenheit and preheat. Spray cooking spray over the baking sheet.
2. Place dried cod filets (after removing excess water) on the baking sheet.
3. Use a small-sized bowl to combine lemon juice and zest, oil, pepper, chili spice, crushed almonds, salt, and dill.
4. Press the filets evenly into mustard (Dijon mustard) with one hand, using the other to divide almond mixture among four filets. Make sure to spread both the sides of filets evenly.
5. Bake for about seven minutes until the thickest portions become opaque.
6. Place the fillets on a plate with vegetables and strips of lemon alongside.

Chapter 7: People's Common Mistakes

Now that you know all about the process of intermittent fasting and how it should be done, you should also have the knowledge of the common mistakes that people make while doing the fast. These mistakes can actually prevent you from realizing the benefits and make the entire fast nothing but a complete waste. So, once you know what they are, make sure that you do not make the same mistakes yourself. If you do not want to make mistakes, the first and foremost thing that you need to do is be aware of everything that you are doing and also know why you are doing them. This will ensure that even if you are sometimes off the path, you can easily push yourself back on track. Also, stop beating yourself up for a cheat day or any mistake that you made. Just move on by accepting that it happened, and it cannot be undone. If you waste your energy in self-loathing, you will not be able to make plans so that the same mistake does not happen twice.

Fasting Too Long Even at the Beginning

You must have heard me saying this plenty of times already; you need to take it slow. Do not rush the process. If you haven't tried intermittent fasting ever in your life, then you should start with a 48-hour fast or even a 24-hour fast for that matter. Yes, you will have to eventually lengthen the fasting window but that does not mean you have to do it now and at once. What you have to do is increase the fasting period but do it in small increments. In case you do not follow what I said, it will be you who will be facing certain consequences and they are bound to happen.

One of the first consequences that people have to face when they fast for longer periods too quickly is that they become grumpy. They behave badly with coworkers and loved ones. And the worst part is that you might shove it away, saying that it's just your way of coping with fasting, but it is not. Also, due to your cranky mood, some people might even give you negative feedback and in most cases, that is when people give up the fast and throw every effort down the gutter all at once. Tossing the whole idea out of the window because of such a situation is not worth it and it would not have come to it only if you had increased your fasting period gradually.

The second consequence is that when people do longer fasts, in the beginning, they cannot continue it after the first couple of days mainly because it becomes too unbearable for them, and they feel tremendously hungry all the time. The process of intermittent fasting should not make you feel jarred or stressed. Instead, it should be gradual and gentle. If you truly want to continue intermittent fasting for a long stretch of time, you have to learn to make it well incorporated into your routine and for that, you need to take it slow. When you start the longer fasts right from the beginning, you are simply walking on the path of disappointment and most people give up too quickly in such cases.

Not Eating the Right Foods

This is probably the biggest mistake that I see people have been making. If you have been trying to incorporate the process of intermittent fasting into your day-to-day life, then you also have to ensure that you are eating the right foods; otherwise, it won't work the way you want it to. For starters, as you might know, fasting means that you have to learn how to get your appetite under control. And this means that you cannot simply grab that packet of chips or that bar of crunchy granola whenever you feel like. There is a time for everything and time is highly essential. But equally essential is what you are eating in your eating window.

If you make the wrong choices, then you are definitely going to have a hard time controlling your appetite. When you are relying on foods that are rich in carbohydrates, you will be deliberately making the entire process difficult for yourself your appetite along with your levels of blood glucose are in a state of continuous fluctuation. When you are on a diet that is low in carbs, you will have more fats and proteins. This will increase your levels of satiety. In simpler words, you will remain full for a longer period of time. Moreover, this will give your body flexibility in metabolism so that you can tap into your fat reserves whenever your body is fasting and does not have enough glucose as fuel.

Also, some people use intermittent fasting as an excuse to eat whatever they want when they are in the eating window. That is not right and won't bring you any good results. You have to remember that this is not a magic pill, and nothing will happen on its own if you do not put enough effort. It is true that intermittent fasting allows you to take your health into your own hands and maintain proper metabolism but for that, your diet needs to be healthy too. You have to cut down on sugar and processed foods. You need to incorporate more and more whole foods that are rich in nutrients and low in carbs.

Consuming Too Many Calories

In the previous point, I told how important it is to eat the right foods so that you can get the nutrients that you need. But at the same time, you should not overdo it in the eating phase. When people fast, they have this idea that they have to replenish themselves by eating an equally heavy meal in the eating window. Never try to compensate for the time you were not eating. Sometimes people end up overeating to such an extent that they not only regret their actions but also feel bloated.

Also, in case you have overeaten, don't be too harsh on yourself because it will only make matters worse. Accept the fact because you simply cannot undo it in any way. What you have to do from now on is that you have to prepare and plan your meals and keep healthy options in every meal. This will ensure that when the eating window starts, you don't have to think about what you want to eat. A very important part of the process of intermittent fasting is to figure out a balance in your routine where you can prepare healthy foods and not depend on processed foods.

Not Staying Consistent

This is probably true for everything on earth that if you are not consistent with it, it will not bring you results. The same goes for intermittent fasting. But what is worse is that if you are not consistent, then you will be stuck in a cycle where you make poor eating choices and you will be so disappointed with everything that you will not feel like doing anything about it. That is exactly something you need to avoid and for this, you have to be consistent. The best way to ensure this is to follow a fasting regime that you can maintain for the long term. You need to understand that if you truly want to reap the benefits of intermittent fasting, then it also means that you have to do it for a long period of time without giving up on it.

In case you already feel like that you will not be able to stay consistent throughout the procedure, then you need to sit down and figure out why. You need to find the reason behind it and then deal with it. Is it because you do not like the method that you have selected? If it is so, then try some other method. Or, is it because your fasting and feeding window is wrong and you are having a hard time adjusting to it? In that case, you need to adjust the timings in a different manner. Whatever it is, just don't give up before figuring out the why.

Doing Too Many Things At the Same Time

This is also one of the reasons why people give up on intermittent fasting, especially beginners. There is a saying that you should not bite off more than you can chew, and this is exactly what I am talking about here. If you are trying out intermittent fasting for the first time and you are also trying to maintain a daily gym schedule (which you don't usually do) and on top that, you are also trying to cook your own meals (when you are habituated to take-outs), then it is very easy to feel stressed.

So, maybe you can start by training only three times a week and then you can take the help of your family members in cooking your meals. If you do not have anyone living with you, then you can skip the gym for now and maybe go for a run in the neighborhood in the initial days. Once you are okay with this routine, then you can incorporate the gym.

Now that you know the common mistakes, I hope this will help you to avoid

Conclusion

Thank you for making it through to the end of *Intermittent Fasting for Women Over 50: Discover How to Lose Weight Fast, Increase Your Energy and Age – Well, Thanks to Intermittent Fasting!,* let's hope it was informative and able to provide you with all of the tools you need to achieve your goals whatever they may be.

Now that you have learned about the process of intermittent fasting, it is time that you start practicing it too. Of late, this subject has gained a lot of attention, and people all over the world have received some amazing results. There are a lot of topics involved in intermittent fasting and if you learn them in-depth, you will realize the processes that go on behind the scenes. If you keep thinking about starting tomorrow, that tomorrow will never come. So, go ahead and start now. Even if it means abstaining from food for a few hours, do it. Then you can work your way up to twelve hours or more. Skip meals and maintain your diet. Do it regularly.

With time, you will realize that you have built the mindset that is required to follow balanced fasting. You will also become aware of the habits that you have inculcated when it comes to diet, and the moment you realize that you will be able to make the healthy shift necessary to maintain good health. Also, it is important that you ease into your fasts and not rush into it. Rushing will only make you impatient and disappointed. Once you fast consistently for about a month or more, you will see the results for yourself and your energy levels will drastically improve.

Finally, if you found this book useful in any way, a review on Amazon is always appreciated!